Start Living, Start Losing

WeightWatchers®

Start Living, Start Losing

Inspirational Stories That Will Motivate You Now

Foreword by Sarah,
Duchess of York

BICENTENNIAL
1807
WILEY
2007
BICENTENNIAL

John Wiley & Sons, Inc.

This book is printed on acid-free paper. ♾

Copyright © 2008 by Weight Watchers. All rights reserved

Published by John Wiley & Sons, Inc., Hoboken, New Jersey
Published simultaneously in Canada

Wiley Bicentennial Logo: Richard J. Pacifico

For general information about our other products and services, please contact our Customer Care Department within the United States at (800) 762–2974, outside the United States at (317) 572–3993 or fax (317) 572–4002.

Wiley also publishes its books in a variety of electronic formats. Some content that appears in print may not be available in electronic books. For more information about Wiley products, visit our web site at www.wiley.com.

Library of Congress Cataloging-in-Publication Data:

Start living, start losing : inspirational stories that will motivate you now / Weight Watchers ; foreword by Sarah, Duchess of York.
   p. cm.
 Includes index.
 ISBN 978-0-470-18914-6 (cloth)
 ISBN 978-1-620-45571-5 (pbk)
 1. Weight loss—Psychological aspects. 2. Motivation (Psychology) I. Weight Watchers International.
 RM222.2.S746 2008
 613.2'5—dc22
   2007039342

Printed in the United States of America

CONTENTS

Foreword by Sarah, Duchess of York

Losing weight is one part organization, one part inspiration. It's one thing to know how to lose weight. Perhaps just as important is a belief that we can—and will.

As you will see in these pages, belief is at the very core of the Weight Watchers experience. Attend any meeting and you cannot help but feel motivated by women and men who have successfully shed weight—and kept it off.

How did they do it? How did *I* do it? I struggled quite famously with my weight for years, flitting from one quick-fix diet to another. In retrospect I fought valiantly, yet ultimately lost the battle because I did not acknowledge what I now know: Diets don't work. And Weight Watchers does. That's because Weight Watchers is not a diet. It's about adopting a healthy lifestyle.

Incredibly, change found me the day I stepped into my first Weight Watchers meeting. All around me were people who were excited about success. Our leader was a glowing success story, of course. But so were the Lifetime Members in the room and also those still working toward their goals.

What I love about this book is that it captures the amazing spirit of a Weight Watchers meeting. I promise you, reading these chapters will motivate you, too!

Everyone loves a dramatic weight-loss story and you have some terrific ones here. No less impressive are the chapters about people whose lives were changed in significant ways by moderate or even modest slimming.

You will see that this collection of personal accounts reminds us that weight-loss success isn't just about losing. It's also about gaining, in terms of better health, improved self-esteem, and a renewed joy for living.

These stories remind us that losing weight can be an empowering, life-changing journey. We often hear that being overweight is a symptom that other things may not be quite right. We see this time and again in these pages, and it's encouraging to see what can happen when mind, body, and soul finally come together in harmony.

I especially like the fact that Weight Watchers has published this book as a celebration of the success that so many of its members enjoy. For all the so-called experts and role models out there who profess to hold the keys to weight loss, isn't it extraordinary that some of the most inspirational figures we'll ever meet are people just like us who are stepping up and winning at the weight game?

There was a time when I felt that my weight was the bane of my existence. Worse, I felt alone in my struggle. My entire life changed, thanks to the sharing and caring I found at Weight Watchers. Provided with the right program and the best support possible from my leader and fellow members, I could not help but succeed.

I think this book's title, *Start Living, Start Losing*, says it all. Make the changes you can live with and you will lose weight. What's more, the experience will transform you from the inside out. I hope you will find inspiration and wisdom in these wonderful stories, as I have.

Acknowledgments

When the editors at Weight Watchers Publishing Group began the process of putting together the manuscript for this book, everyone we approached was enthusiastic about the assignment. We began to build a team that spanned the United States and included real people who graciously shared their stories and a group of talented writers, editors, and designers who brought these stories to life. Soon that enthusiasm grew, spurring an even greater commitment and passion. We wanted to make sure we told stories in each individual's voice to capture the scope of events and emotions that occur when a person is trying to lose weight or lead a healthier life. Many people need to be acknowledged for their efforts, as well as for their dedication. The individuals who shared their stories are to be thanked for their time and heartfelt honesty. The editorial group was led by editor and writer Stacey Colino, whose skill and commitment were a guiding force for the writing team of Emma Smith, Ginny Graves, Kathleen Doheny, Elinor Nauen, and Sheryl Berk. Many thanks are also extended to members of Weight Watchers Publishing Group who made invaluable contributions, including Jennifer Matarazzo, Celia Shatzman, and Ed Melnitsky. Special thanks to Maura McEvoy for capturing a spirit and joy in her photos and to Tom Miller, our editor at Wiley, who provided a skilled guiding hand in making the manuscript a richer read for all.

—Nancy Gagliardi
Editorial Director
Weight Watchers Publishing Group

Introduction

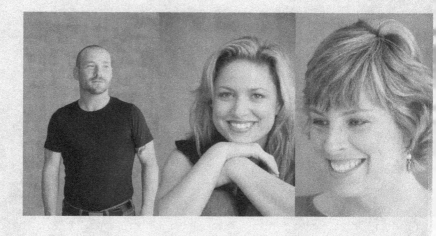

Everyone loves a loser—that is, someone who has succeeded at losing weight. For more than forty years, Weight Watchers, a highly respected name in weight management, has been helping millions of people do just that: lose weight and reclaim a healthier life. Weight Watchers is acknowledged by health-care professionals and organizations worldwide as a trusted source of science-based information about healthy eating, physical activity, and behavior modification. A 2007 survey conducted by Double Helix Development asked doctors who recommended structured weight-loss programs to their patients which specific programs they recommended. Almost two-thirds of those doctors recommended Weight Watchers.

More people have come to Weight Watchers to lose weight and keep it off than have tried any other commercial weight-loss plan. With this in mind, Weight Watchers is opening its doors to share with you some of the most powerful success stories of people who've lost weight on the Weight Watchers program, maintained that loss, and changed their lives. We combed through thousands of stories—some submitted by Weight Watchers members, others referred by their leaders, and still others heard of through the Weight Watchers grapevine as "a great story." The fact is, there are thousands of great stories. So after sorting and interviewing and writing and more interviewing, we've compiled a series of diverse stories. With them, we hope to inspire you to strive toward your weight and health goals and to create a healthier lifestyle that you can maintain in the long run.

While we were compiling this collection of stories, we noted several recurring thoughts or revelations as the members spoke about their experiences (and results) on the Weight Watchers program. We noted four distinct themes that we want to share because they provide universal clues that can help you on the road to achieving your own personal success.

- **I Need to Change.** The first theme we found in many of the success stories revolves around that one moment each person has when he or she truly decides to lose the weight for good. This moment tends to result from an unexpected event or emotion that jolts the person to say, "I need to make a change." Many of these Aha! moments transcend demographics. Whether it's seeing his or her image on a video from a family wedding, hearing a family physician deliver the results of a medical test, or watching a loved one battle a weight-related illness, when that moment arrives, something triggers the person to take action.

- **I Can Do It.** When someone finally walks through the doors and into a Weight Watchers meeting, that individual meets a variety of people from all walks of life, which helps him or her to realize that anyone can follow the plan. This is another key revelation we found throughout the stories. People featured in these Weight Watchers success stories range in age from twenty to seventy; they hail from across the United States, as well as around the globe. Some have 10 pounds to lose; others, 100. Their lives and experiences are diverse, whether it's a truck driver from New Jersey, a credit bureau account specialist from Texas, or a home-schooling mother of four from Kansas. Yet they are bound by the fact that anyone can follow the program and get results.

- **I Need to Create a Supportive Environment.** Another theme that resonates in all of these success stories is that a supportive environment is crucial when it comes to achieving your weight-loss goals and, most important, keeping the weight off for the long haul. One example of that supportive environment is Weight Watchers meetings. In fact, research published in the May 2004 supplement to the *International Journal of Obesity* found that 80 percent of the weight lost by people who followed the Weight Watchers plan during both their weight-loss and maintenance phases was maintained after one year. This contrasts sharply with a 1992 National Institutes of Health (NIH) expert panel's consensus statement, which, after evaluating a variety of programs and methods, concluded that a person completing a weight-loss program can expect to keep only 33 percent of the weight off after a year. This 2004 study is important, we think, for two reasons: not only does it demonstrate the importance of a livable program combined with support, but it also puts to rest the idea that all weight-loss programs yield the same results.

- **I Changed My Life.** A final recurring theme apparent within these stories is that once members have achieved success and reached their goals, the rewards are many and, in many ways, life changing. From an increase in energy and a boost in confidence to the reversal of diseases such as diabetes and hypertension and the rediscovery of a "former self," Weight Watchers members recognize how dramatically their lives are altered by having reached their goals.

As you read the stories in *Start Living, Start Losing*, these four themes will come up again and again in the voices and words of your sisters and brothers, your friends, neighbors, and colleagues, even celebrities. The stories reveal in compelling, poignant, and sometimes humorous detail members' experiences of slimming down. For example, in "Scared Serious," you will read about Rolando, forty-one, who got his wake-up call to lose weight after suffering chest pains. There's also Dawn, thirty-eight, in "Losing Weight, Finding My Sisters," who decided to lose weight after signing up for a marathon to raise money for leukemia in memory of a sister who had died of the disease. And in "Bouncing Back after Baby," funny lady Jenny McCarthy, thirty-six, will have you laughing with her graphic descriptions of how her body changed after she had a baby and what she did to get her pre-baby body back.

You will read stories that chronicle personal frustrations, challenges, and triumphs. Feeling stuck—physically, emotionally, or metaphorically—is at the heart of many stories because being overweight had prevented these women and men from doing things they really wanted to do with their lives. Often, it isn't the excess weight itself but the impact on one's confidence and self-esteem that causes people to feel stuck. In "Keeping a Sense of Humor," Bettyann, fifty-eight, describes the shame she felt at not being able to fit through the turnstiles at her beloved Mets games or to sit in regular theater seats. In "Finding Me Again," Stacey, forty, shares the story of how she overcame her perceptions that she couldn't get out of an unhappy marriage or become a fitness instructor because she was overweight. And in "Acting My Way to Weight Loss," Shuler, forty, a Broadway actor, reveals how he reached the decision to shed pounds in order to become more agile on stage and to change the way he suspected that his children saw him.

In reading these stories, you'll get a bird's-eye view of the factors that contributed to these people's weight and their relationship with food and how they felt about their bodies. You'll gain an intimate glimpse at what triggered their desire to lose, how they were able to set their plans in motion, and what they did to overcome roadblocks and obstacles along the way. You will learn from those who have found success. Finally, you'll cheer them on as you read about the turning points they experienced when they realized just how far they'd come in their journeys toward thin and how they changed internally along the way.

These are people who didn't quit. They persevered, found, and—perhaps most important—maintained their success. They learned from the mistakes they made and found ways to fix them. They discovered—through trial and error and with the help of the supportive environment they created—how to keep going after they hit weight plateaus or faced new challenges. After all, their stories also address practical considerations: how to incorporate your favorite foods into your life without gaining again, how to fit exercise into an already hectic schedule, and how to fill up with convenient, healthy snacks throughout the day, among many others.

Ultimately, you'll discover what they see as the biggest payoffs of becoming lighter and what they learned about themselves as they tackled and embraced this life-enhancing transformation. In all likelihood, these insights will change the way you view the weight-loss journey. Whether you read the stories in this book sequentially or come back to them again and again when you need a dose of inspiration, *Start Living, Start Losing* is sure to motivate you to launch—or support you as you continue—your own plan for healthy living.

CHAPTER 1

Mirror, Mirror

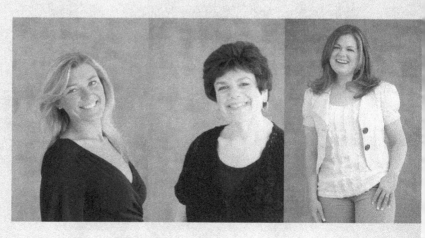

For many people, losing weight is about being able to dress the way they want or simply liking the way their bodies look. For others, it's about coming out of hiding and showing themselves to the world. In this chapter, you'll hear from men and women who spent years struggling with poor body esteem or feeling uncomfortable in their own skin—and who then took action to change those feelings by changing their habits. As they talk about how their weight struggles affected the way they felt about themselves, you'll realize just how universal body-image issues are. You'll also be inspired to tackle your own feelings about how you look.

Size Matters

Kristy, 37, California, bookkeeper

All through high school, I wasn't really heavy—I was a size 12 or 14, what I think of as a normal size because I'm tall. I'm 5 feet 8 inches. In terms of weight, I was in the middle, between people who are really small and those who are very big—and I was pretty much okay with that.

Then I got married in my early twenties and I started gaining weight, about 40 pounds. It wasn't like I got married and decided to relax my eating habits, though I did start eating doughnuts a lot. My husband began to work out of town and wasn't home much. So I ate out a lot—and too much fast food. I went up to a size 16, which wasn't normal for me.

We got divorced a year and a half after we were married. I was so upset, and the weight just came off. I was back to my usual size 12 or 14. I was so devastated about the divorce that I couldn't even be happy about the weight loss. But about six months later, after I had adjusted to being a divorced mom, I was happy to be a normal size again.

Then, in August 2004, my dad died. He had cancer so it wasn't that he died suddenly. We knew it was coming. He and I weren't very close, and I guess I didn't think it would affect me as much as it did. But I put on 30 pounds in the months after he died. Even with the excess weight, I think I was in denial about how I looked. I still had this image of myself from before—that I was still pretty normal.

Then I got a very rude awakening. Gayle, one of my best friends, got married in Vegas in February 2005. It was a second wedding for her, and it was just me standing up for her. When the pictures came back, Gayle wanted to show them to me right away. I took a look, and my face must have registered anything but happiness for her because she asked me what the matter was. To tell you the truth, I was taken by surprise. Yes, I was happy for her, but I couldn't believe how bad I looked in the pictures. I was dressed up nice, with a cute dress, and my hair was fixed, but I thought that it just didn't look like me. I looked so heavy!

Worse, I was standing next to one of the guys in the wedding party and I felt like I kind of eclipsed him because I was so big. And that's not normal; usually, the guy is bigger. I don't want to be bigger than guys. I'm already bigger than some because I am tall so I don't want to be heavier, too.

That's when I knew I had to get serious about losing weight. One of the other mothers at my son's school had lost weight by going to Weight Watchers. So at the end of February 2005, I joined and weighed in at 193 pounds. I knew I had a lot of work to do.

I lost 43 pounds over the next five months by taking a hard look at my eating habits. I started eating a sensible breakfast and going home from the office for lunch so I could fix a turkey or chicken sandwich on wheat bread and have some sugar-free strawberry Jell-O if my sweet tooth kicked up. I drank a ton of water, sometimes close to a gallon a day. I love to eat dinner out, but I stopped doing it as often. While trying to lose, I also began to exercise, mostly on the treadmill, and I discovered that I actually enjoy it.

At one point, I got down to 146 pounds, which was below my goal, but it was too much of a struggle to maintain. I felt as if I didn't get enough to eat when I tried to stay at that weight. I felt tired and hungry a lot of the time. And I just don't have that much willpower to be so good all the time.

Now, my weight ranges between 155 and 160—I am more comfortable there and it's still healthy. This now feels like a normal weight for me, and most of the time I feel pretty good about how I look. But sometimes I see thin girls who are wolfing down big burgers, and they look like they don't have a care in the world—and I have a little twinge of jealousy.

But I know that's not realistic or even normal for most people. And I've come to terms with the fact that I'm never going to be a size 4. My ancestors are Samoan and German so I'm a big-boned girl. The good thing is, at my current weight, I know I'm a lot healthier than I used to be.

Even after losing weight, I still focus a lot on the size issue, though now it's often in a good way. Recently, I bought a pair of size-8 pants, which means I'm three sizes skinnier than what I used to consider normal for me. It feels great. I guess what's normal is all relative.

TAKE-AWAY: Start your day with a sensible breakfast

Not only will eating a morning meal jump-start your energy for the day, but it can help you to avoid overeating at lunch-time and will keep your mood on a more even keel.

A Transforming Experience

Kimberla Lawson Roby, 42, Illinois, *New York Times* best-selling novelist

I decided to lose weight in May 2005 because I had just turned forty and realized it was high time I started taking better care of myself. I was beginning to feel tired all the time, even after a full night's rest. And I was truly tired of all the yo-yo dieting I'd been doing for years, to no avail. Every time I would try to lose weight on one fad diet after another, I'd always end up gaining every pound back and then some. I was riding a very vicious and frustrating cycle. I finally decided enough was enough.

In addition, my weight was affecting my career. The extra pounds made me feel as though I didn't look or feel as good as I could have. Whenever I would head out on national book tours or travel to individual speaking engagements, I was always concerned about what clothing I would wear and how it probably wasn't going to fit properly or look as presentable as I wanted it to. Because my eating habits were terrible, I couldn't resist ordering room service at hotels late at night; then I'd go to sleep on a full stomach, feeling miserable. But the worst thing of all was the fact that I was always exhausted on every trip I took. I just didn't feel as energized as I should have.

"I eat a wide variety of foods—I love baked fish, particularly salmon and walleye, partly because it tastes so good and partly because it's very healthy."

After I joined Weight Watchers, I attended meetings every single week without fail, no matter what I had scheduled for Thursday afternoons. The meetings really helped me to keep up my motivation. I even attended one in New York while my husband and I were there, celebrating our fifteenth wedding anniversary.

While I was losing, my husband was one of my biggest cheerleaders. He supported my decision to join Weight Watchers from the very first moment I mentioned it. And my best friends Kelli and Lori encouraged me daily. It also helped that I made my weight-loss efforts my top priority this time, and I rewarded myself for losing. Whenever I went down a size, I went shopping and treated myself to a new pair of jeans that actually fit.

My biggest challenge was cutting back on sweets because I do love them so! I still love chocolate and pizza, but now I indulge in sensible moderation. While losing weight, I stopped overeating and ate only enough to feel satisfied. Today, I eat a wide variety of foods—I love baked fish, particularly salmon and walleye, partly because it tastes so good and partly because it's very healthy—but the difference is that I consume much, much smaller portions than I did during my pre–Weight Watchers days.

The other major change is that I began working out on a regular basis. Now I walk thirty to forty minutes per day, either on a treadmill or on a bike path, and I tone with weights two to three times per week. These days, I love my arms—they are more toned than ever before.

I realized I'd reached a turning point with my weight the day I learned that I'd lost my first 10 pounds. I was so excited to be having great success—and I wasn't feeling hungry or discontented. It was then that I knew I could go all the way. And I did: I've now lost 40 pounds in total on my own and through Weight Watchers.

The best thing about being thinner is that I feel so much more energized and a lot more limber. I feel better today than I did in my late twenties or early thirties. While slimming down, I learned that it really is possible to look and feel a lot younger than you actually are. Every day, I remind myself that this is a wonderfully healthy lifestyle change, one that has transformed my life physically, spiritually, and emotionally.

TAKE-AWAY: Avoid eating a big meal late at night

Going to sleep with a full stomach can compromise the quality of your sleep and leave you feeling sluggish and uncomfortable the next morning.

My New Neck

Sharon, 55, New Jersey, Weight Watchers training manager

I was a member of Weight Watchers for many years before I lost weight for good. I'd join and lose some weight and quit, then I would rejoin and lose again and quit, and so on. My gradual weight gain started in college, but I just ignored it, until it continued to get worse after I was married. I was on and off Weight Watchers for years before I finally made up my mind to really commit to it.

That was in 1979, and I rejoined because I knew I wanted to have a baby and I didn't want to gain weight on top of the extra weight I was already carrying. I made this a priority, and I decided I had to treat losing weight like a pregnancy, so I gave it nine months. I would not miss meetings because the minute I missed the meetings, I had a bad week. I'd think I was on a little break so I'd give in to whatever I'd been having a yen for and I'd end up overeating. Finally, I learned that coming to the meetings put a stop to the mess-ups. It took me ten months to lose 50 pounds, and I found out that I was pregnant the week I reached my goal. Shortly after that, I started working for Weight Watchers, and now I'm a training manager.

I'm very proud of the fact that I've maintained my weight loss for twenty-five years. I think a lot of people assume that once they've reached their goal weight they're cured and can go back to their regular lives. But I learned tricks to keep the weight off. For example, I used to have bad nails, but I started to polish them every evening to use that as a way not to eat at night. I like my new body, and it's the same idea—I want to continue to look good so I know I need to continue some of the healthy habits I've learned, like controlling portion sizes.

I felt so much better after I lost weight, but the part I never lost was my neck. I always had a double chin, and when I looked in the mirror, I still had the heavy face, the heavy neck. It was just kind of hanging there. I always said that if I ever had money, I would do something about it.

In 1997, a friend who had had cosmetic surgery offered to go with me for a consultation with a plastic surgeon. When computer imaging showed what I could look like, I said, "Oh my gosh . . . that looks great!" But I have four kids, and when I heard the price I said, "There's no way." I just couldn't justify it.

About a year later I was left some money by my best friend, Janet, who died of breast cancer. Before she died, she said to me, "Now I don't want you to use this on the kids or the house. This is for you." I felt as if she had just shown me how short life was, so I decided to do it.

When I finally went for the surgery, it was just before my forty-seventh birthday. The surgeon suggested that I have my eyelids done, too. He lifted my lids, then he lifted my neck by cutting underneath and behind my ears and pulling up just the neck part. I felt a lot of discomfort the first two days after surgery, but I had thought it was going to be much more painful so I was pleasantly surprised.

"I think a lot of people assume that once they've reached their goal weight they're cured and can go back to their regular lives. But I learned tricks to keep the weight off."

Having the surgery has made me feel so much happier. I was always confident, but when I'd look at pictures of myself, I would feel disappointed because I would only see my sagging neck. I couldn't really focus on the rest of me. I feel so good when I look at pictures now.

Everybody asks me whether it was worth it. I really think it was. It made me feel really good about myself, and that was important at that stage in my life. After taking care of kids all my life, it was my turn.

TAKE-AWAY: Polish your nails in the evening

If you do something with your hands—such as giving yourself a manicure or doing needlepoint or knitting—you'll make it impossible to snack after dinner; plus, you'll distract yourself from the desire to do so.

On Campus and Still Losing

Caryn, 20, Pennsylvania, college student

I was overweight at a young age, but halfway through my freshman year of college, I hit my all-time high. At home, my mom cooked balanced meals, but at school, my options were mostly pizza, cheeseburgers, french fries, ice cream, chips, candy, anything deep-fried. My first semester, I ate anything I wanted and was having a lot of fun—until I took a step back and saw that I had gained 30 pounds in four months! It was just too much drinking and partying and living off the fatty foods at the campus dining halls. My weight hit almost 190 pounds. I am 5 feet 3 inches.

I wanted to wear hip clothes like my classmates, but low-rise jeans just don't look as great when your belly is hanging over the waistband. I felt uncomfortable in my own skin and was low on self-confidence. It got to the point where I would cry about how I looked, but because I have been overweight for most of my life, I just assumed that was who I was and nothing would change it.

One night, I was watching a marathon of *The Biggest Loser* on TV. Seeing those people who were way bigger than me change their lives and become the skinny person that I always wanted to be—well, it just hit me and I thought, "I can do that, too!" That's when I joined Weight Watchers. From that first meeting in February 2006, my battle with weight seemed so much easier. Hearing other people's stories and advice made me feel like everything I was going through was normal.

"My dorm room became my kitchen. For breakfast, I would buy fat-free yogurt, fruit, and high-fiber cereal and keep that in my room. For lunch, maybe I'd make a sandwich in my room."

But I had a lot of challenges back at school. Eating at the dining halls, going out to dinner with friends who never had to diet, and living in a dorm room with no kitchen did not make losing easy. But I had to make it work. Basically, my dorm room became my kitchen. For breakfast, I would buy fat-free yogurt, fruit, and high-fiber cereal and keep that in my room. For lunch, maybe I'd make a sandwich in my room. I ate most dinners in restaurants and learned a good lesson in how to be assertive with waiters: I'd often ask them to prepare something special for me. The way I see it, I'm paying for the food, and it is important that it be prepared in a healthy way.

Going out and drinking with my friends became another obstacle. Let's face it: I didn't want to hurt my social life, but I did want to lose weight. So at first I'd save up a few ***POINTS*®** for a drink. But after a while it seemed silly to waste empty calories on alcohol so I'd just sip on a diet soda. No one could even tell it had no alcohol in it, and it made me fit in more just to be holding a cup. To tell you the truth, I have so much fun watching other people get drunk and doing silly things.

So far, I've lost 60 pounds. Once I started losing weight, I began to look at my whole life and food differently. Now I eat to live, not live to eat. I still sometimes overeat, but there's no way I'm going to throw away what I've worked so hard for. Now, if I mess up, I just get rid of the junk food and start fresh.

TAKE-AWAY: Be assertive when dining out
Quiz your waiter about how a dish is prepared, and don't be shy about asking the chef to prepare something without sauces or extra fat. These days, many chefs are willing to do just that.

Wearing My Daughter's Clothes

Dee, 55, Georgia, receptionist and Weight Watchers meeting leader

Even as a child I was always one of the bigger kids in the class, but I never really thought of myself as fat. I'd say I was *fluffy*—that was my word. Fluffy sounds a lot better than fat. But as an adult I gained about 5 pounds a year, and by the time I was in my late forties, I was getting pretty tired of being overweight. My knees were aching, and my back and my ankles, too. My husband and I went to my daughter's high school graduation in 2001, and when I looked around at the other mothers, I felt as if I looked like a grandmother. They were all wearing these cute, hip clothes, and I was wearing old lady stuff—matronly stuff—because of my weight. That made me mad. I thought, "I can't do anything about my age, but I can certainly do something about my size."

One day my daughter was looking for something to wear because she was going out that night, and she was begging me to buy her something new. I told her she had plenty of lovely clothes, some brand-new with the tags still on. So I decided to go fishing through her closet and find her something to wear. She caught me in there and said, "What are you doing?" I said, "Look at all these beautiful clothes! I'd kill to be able to wear them." She said, "Momma, you could if you'd lose about 100 pounds."

Well, let me tell you, that was like a slap in the face, but it was the best slap I ever got. I thought, "I'm going to show her. I will lose 100 pounds."

I weighed 242 pounds when I joined. That was in September 2001—the 13th, just two days after 9/11. The timing motivated me, too. I thought, "So many people didn't even make it to this day. I'm going to take better care of myself from now on."

In one of the first meetings, the leader explained that obesity could contribute to cancer. That was a total surprise to me. I had been treated for breast cancer the year before, and I thought, "*There's* another reason to lose weight. I'm going to get this weight off because I don't ever want to go through that again." Breast cancer was scary, and I really didn't want it to come back.

I also started to wonder whether my poor eating habits were part of the reason I got cancer. I was kind of like a junk-food junkie. I ate fast food, cookies, potato chips, candy bars, and if I ate a real meal, it was all fried foods and starch. But my favorite was cake, especially red velvet cake. It has this creamy frosting with nuts on it. It's the greatest thing there is. If I got hold of a red velvet cake, I'd have cake for breakfast, cake for a snack, cake for lunch, and cake for dinner. I would even wake up in the middle of the night and swear that cake was calling my name and I'd go get a piece. I wasn't in control of food; food was in control of me.

So getting started was a big adjustment. When they told me I should try to drink forty-eight ounces of water a day, I was like, "*'Scuse* me? I don't drink forty-eight ounces of water in a month!" I couldn't do it initially. I had at best two glasses a day, but over time I worked my way up. And all those fruits and vegetables? Oh, brother. I had never really eaten them before. But I found that I liked cabbage and salad, and I kept pushing myself to try new things. Now I like just about any kind of vegetable, but it took me a good long while to get there.

> "When they told me I should try to drink forty-eight ounces of water a day, I was like, '*Scuse* me? I don't drink forty-eight ounces of water in a month!' I couldn't do it initially. I had at best two glasses a day, but over time I worked my way up."

I lost about a pound a week. I wasn't willing to do anything super strict because I figured that would never work anyway. My daughter was a great support. If she knew I wanted some dessert or something, she'd say, "Momma, you can have it, but maybe we should split it." The other thing that really helped me stick with the program—and helps me to this day—is loving how I look when I'm thinner. Early on, my meeting leader said it helps to have a goal, so I decided to try to lose 50 pounds by the time I turned fifty, which was about seven months away at that point. I was going to throw myself a birthday party and call it "Fine and Foxy at Fifty." I didn't quite make that goal—I was a few pounds shy—but I was still fine and foxy when I turned fifty.

About six months after starting Weight Watchers, I began to walk two miles every day. I had never exercised before, but I really enjoyed it. I found that it was a great way to relieve stress, and it made me feel healthier. I reached my goal of 164 in December 2002, and I've stayed a little below that ever since. I'm a size 10, so I can wear clothes that are fun and hip—even some of my daughter's.

I recently attended her college graduation, and when I looked around at the other mothers, I didn't feel like a grandmother anymore. I looked like a mother—and a hot one at that!

TAKE-AWAY: Push yourself to try at least one new fruit or vegetable per week

You'll be treating yourself to a new taste sensation and a variety of nutrients—and you'll be helping to expand your culinary repertoire in a healthy, low-calorie way.

Looking Suitable

Fred, 65, Illinois, attorney

When I was a child, I had a book called the *Wonder Book of Knowledge*. In it was a story about Egypt, and there was a picture of King Farouk, the last monarch, standing in a swimsuit on a beach somewhere. He was a corpulent man, and the picture wasn't very flattering. I remember thinking, "Gee, I hope I never look like that." Well, one morning, I looked in the mirror and saw King Farouk. It bothered me immensely.

I had recently received a significant promotion at work—I was made the head of a governmental law department—and I didn't think the image I portrayed was appropriate for the office. In my new position, I had to appear before a board of nine elected commissioners and speak from a rostrum. One day it occurred to me that being as heavy as I was reflected a personal disregard. I felt slovenly, even though I was neatly dressed. That wasn't the image I wanted to portray. Also, most of my colleagues were thinner than I was, and I felt that being overweight signified a loss of control and a lack of confidence.

Since it was January, my wife and I were making our annual resolutions. Every year we resolved that we would lose weight and start exercising, and every year we did nothing. But after my King Farouk experience, we decided to join Weight Watchers. We did it as sort of a lark because nothing had ever worked for me. We went to the first meeting with another couple, and we cut up quite a bit. I think the leader was sort of upset with us because we weren't taking it seriously. But our attitude changed very quickly when I saw that it worked. I weighed 263 pounds when we started, and the weight started to come off right away.

I don't think I would have stuck with it if my wife hadn't done it with me. We both had to shift our habits significantly. She is an excellent cook, but she had a habit of cooking large portions. She had to learn to cook smaller quantities, and I needed to cut down on the amount of food I ate. That part was difficult. As a child I was told, "Clean your plate, there are hungry children in China." I followed that warning and cleaned my plate; then I'd fill it up and clean it again. That approach didn't do me any favors.

I forced myself to stop taking seconds—and to stop snacking after dinner or at least to have better snacks. I love salty food, so for a long time my exclusive snack was a small bag of pretzel thins. I also bought a treadmill and started to walk 2.5 miles a night. As I got more fit, I picked up the pace and added some mileage. It's just part of my regimen now. When we're on vacation, we always look for hotels with exercise rooms.

> "I bought a treadmill and started to walk 2.5 miles a night. As I got more fit, I picked up the pace and added some mileage. It's just part of my regimen now. When we're on vacation, we always look for hotels with exercise rooms."

In January 2007, almost a year to the day from the time I started, I reached my goal of 190. My wife was still a ways from her goal, but she was very happy for me because she had been concerned about my weight.

Now my clothes fit well, and I wear flashier suits. In my heavier state, my clothing was always somber—I wore dark blue or black suits. Now I wear pastel or even red shirts and some jewelry, like a gold bracelet and a gold wristwatch. The colors and the style seem to suit my position better. My clothing and my slim physique convey confidence and authority—almost a little swagger. Now when I'm standing at the rostrum, I'm dressing and looking the part—and I'm feeling it, too. I feel better about myself, and I think my employers have more confidence in me.

The last time my wife and I went shopping, I couldn't find a suit that fit right because I needed a 48 jacket and 38 pants. We discovered these athletic-cut suits that looked very nice. The woman who was helping us said, "I generally sell these suits to younger men. No one over fifty buys them." But they fit me perfectly. When I looked in the mirror, I was very pleased with my image. King Farouk was nowhere in sight.

TAKE-AWAY: Quit the clean plate club

If you get out of the habit of finishing what's on your plate—and stop eating when you're pleasantly satisfied, instead—you'll spare yourself loads of unnecessary calories at every meal.

From Overweight Mom to Fit Triathlete

Rina, 43, California, art teacher

I can still remember the ad I put in our community paper, word for word:

> *Forty-year-old mom seeks high school athlete to train her for an upcoming fall triathlon. Must be able to run, bike, and swim 5 hours a week. $8.50 an hour.*

The ad sounded like some fit suburban mom, just trying to save on a personal trainer. But I was forty, out of shape, and about 30 pounds overweight. I wasn't an athlete. I'd never even thought about entering a triathlon—until I got a holiday photo from my old friend Anne-Marie.

Like me, she was forty. Like me, she had two kids. But Anne-Marie had always been fit and never had a weight problem. In the photo, she still didn't have a weight problem: the picture was of Anne-Marie and her husband in workout clothes. The letter that came with the photo said they had taken up triathlons. She looked amazing—radiant, beautiful, happy.

Pretty much the opposite of me. I was fat, unhappy, dowdy, stressed out. I wasn't exercising. The year before, my husband and I and our two boys had moved from Texas to California. The move was a big stress; we had problems every which way. I gave up my job as an art teacher in Texas and started studying to get licensed in California. I didn't have friends here yet. It seems that whenever I sat down at the computer, which was often, I was also eating.

Looking at that photo of Anne-Marie jolted me out of my funk. I heard myself say, "If she can do it, I can do it." I went online and found a triathlon nearby later in the year. I registered for it. I felt really pumped up and told everyone about it because I knew that if I went public, I couldn't let myself fail.

Pretty soon, the reality hit me: I needed to train for this event. It included a 500-meter swim, a 15-kilometer bike ride, and a 5-kilometer run. That's when I knew I had to hire a coach. Personal trainers are expensive, but high school kids always want to make money. So I put the ad in the paper, trying to find a high school athlete who could help me. A local kid on the lacrosse and football teams answered my ad. His name was Will. We started training on Mother's Day 2004, first focusing on the running (I barely jogged!). We ran a minute, walked a minute, ran a minute, walked a minute. By the tenth minute, I lay down in the dirt and nearly passed out.

Eventually, I got up. And we kept on training. I knew my weight was working against me, but it was a difficult time to try to lose. So my weight just kept going up and up. I went up to 147, too much for my small frame—I'm 5 feet ½ inch.

> "We ran a minute, walked a minute, ran a minute, walked a minute. By the tenth minute, I lay down in the dirt and nearly passed out. Eventually, I got up.

One day when I was on my computer, an ad popped up for Weight Watchers Online. I knew it would be easier for me to run if I was lighter so I signed up then and there. Being an online subscriber was perfect for me, since I had my two young children at home.

The first two months, I lost 8 pounds. The weight came off slowly, but the more I lost, the easier my training became. I was jazzed. After five months, I hit my goal of losing 10 percent of my weight. By June 2005, I got down to my goal, 118. I never thought I'd ever be less than 120 pounds again.

But then again, I never thought I would be crossing the finish line of a triathlon. And that's what I did in October 2004. I was last in my age group, but who cares? The most exciting part of the race was seeing the finish line. When I saw the word "Finish," it was one of the happiest moments of my life.

TAKE-AWAY: Say yes to a worthy challenge

Instead of automatically saying no to activities or events that sound difficult or time-consuming, accept the challenge of doing something that's healthy for you physically and emotionally; it'll be good for your weight as well as your state of mind.

Waving Good-bye
to Excuses

Christine, 40, Michigan, director of library services

My weight has gone up and down for pretty much my whole life. Everyone in my family is overweight so I just thought, "The metabolism gods are against me." Even at my heaviest, I was probably 100 pounds less than anyone in my family. It really started in middle school—that's when I got heavy. Then I was thin in high school, but I gained weight my freshman year in college. When I got married at twenty-four, I weighed 152—I'm almost 5 feet 8 inches—and I wore a size 8. But then I gained 5 or more pounds every year until I got pregnant with my daughter five years later. For a while, my weight stayed around 175 or 180, except for when I was pregnant with my two kids.

In the back of my mind, I thought that someday I'd lose weight, but I didn't have a whole lot of time for myself. I was a walking zombie when my kids were young, and I wasn't getting enough sleep. Plus, I had all kinds of excuses: I don't have time to work out; I'm too busy; it's my poor metabolism or the way my family is built. I told myself, "I have just a little weight to lose; it's no big deal."

But finally, those extra pounds really started to bother me. I had gained about 5 more pounds and my size 12s were just so, so tight on me. It was a really hot summer, and I was very uncomfortable. I've always been an exerciser, and I started walking seven days a week to try to lose weight, but I only lost 3 pounds in two months. In July, we went to visit a couple in Sweden whom we'd met on our honeymoon. When we'd first gotten acquainted, the woman and I were pretty much the same size; at one point, she'd gained weight and done Weight Watchers in Sweden, and she told me it was so easy.

While we were over there, we took pictures and I was pretty embarrassed because I'd gained enough weight that you could really see it in my face and my arms. But when we got home and I saw the side view of myself in candid shots that were taken by someone else, it was quite shocking to realize how bad I really looked. I thought, "This is ridiculous!" Finally, I made a decision that I'd had enough of it. No more excuses! I started trying to lose weight within a week after returning from Europe.

I signed up for Weight Watchers Online. I work full time and then some—three people had my job a few years ago—and we have two kids, who are now eleven and nine. My husband is a teacher and a coach so we are busy every night. As it is, I have to get up at 5 a.m. to exercise so the online plan fit into my lifestyle.

It wasn't until I started trying to lose weight that I realized where I was going wrong—and I really wasn't going that wrong. I just needed to learn a little bit more, mostly about portion control. Even though I was eating healthy foods, I needed to eat less of them and eat more fruits and vegetables. My husband is extremely thin—he is 6 feet 2 inches, weighs 180, and can pretty much eat whatever he wants to and I'll gain the weight. So he eats huge portions and all kinds of desserts to try to keep his weight up—and I was eating those things, too. That had to change. Now, rather than having a side dish of broccoli, I'll put a huge serving of broccoli on my plate and half a hamburger on the side. That's helped me to feel full and cut down on calories. At school, kids are constantly bringing around birthday treats so I used to have a cupcake and think it was just a little snack. After starting the plan, I realized it should be more like a once-a-week treat, not a daily one. Keeping a journal and being more cognizant of my eating habits really helped.

> "Now, rather than having a side dish of broccoli, I'll put a huge serving of broccoli on my plate and half a hamburger on the side. That's helped me to feel full and cut down on calories."

It took me two and a half months to reach my first goal, then I ended up resetting my goal two more times. Initially, I thought I just needed to lose about 20 pounds, and when I reached that, I thought I looked horrible so I reset my goal to 150. Then, when I reached that, I thought I still looked heavy so I reset my goal to 135. When I got to 135, I still had a flabby stomach and I hated it, but I decided that I need to be realistic—I'm never going to look like Cindy Crawford—so now I pretty much stay at 133.

Losing weight has given me a lot more confidence in how I look, but I'm still the very same person inside. I don't mind people asking me how I lost weight if they're interested in losing weight, but I really don't like it when people, especially men, make comments to me about how I look. My neighbor came up to me at his daughter's graduation party and said, "Boy, you're hot!" right in front of his eighteen-year-old daughter and my husband. I've actually had quite a bit of that—and it makes me pretty uncomfortable. Other people have made comments to me like, "Boy, I'll bet your husband is just so happy that you've lost weight!"—and I was offended by that because my husband always loved me just the way I was. I never felt like I had to do it for him.

I'm glad that I lost weight, but I did it for me, not for anyone else. We have a swimming pool and people like to come over and go swimming; I used to feel very uncomfortable being in a bathing suit around them. Now I'm much more comfortable and confident in the way I look. That was important for my own self-esteem. Now I feel good about myself, inside and outside.

TAKE-AWAY: View sweet treats realistically

If you want to lose weight, you can't have high-calorie sweets—cakes, cookies, candy, or full-fat ice cream—whenever you feel like it. You need to either find a lower-calorie substitute that you can have every day or save the rich desserts for once a week.

Show Yourself Signs of Success

Success breeds success. To help yourself maintain your motivation or your newly slimmer status, display a picture of yourself that you love or a certificate of what you've accomplished in a place where you'll see it regularly. What other ways can you sing your own praises?

_____

_____

_____

_____

_____

_____

_____

_____

_____

_____

_____

CHAPTER 2

Family Matters

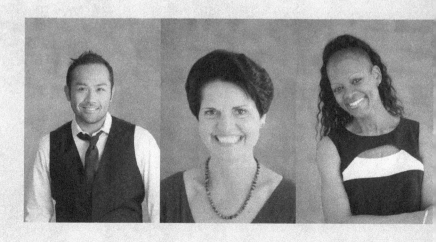

Having a family means never having to eat alone. It also means there's a good chance your habits will have a ripple effect on others. Coming to this realization inspires many overweight people to make lifestyle changes that will help them to slim down. The men and the women featured in this chapter share their struggles to balance work and family responsibilities, while shedding unhealthy habits. Their stories will motivate you and provide you with ideas on how you can be a role model for your clan while losing weight.

Making Time for Me

Elizabeth, 43, Ohio, attorney and court manager

I am a highly organized person. I live on a schedule and have a list for absolutely everything. I even typeset my grocery list so that all I have to do is circle what we need every time I shop. In fact, to keep track of everything I have going on, I keep a computerized, detailed calendar that I print out and then add to as needed. I'd be sunk if I didn't have my calendar or my lists.

I'm an attorney and I work full time. I have a husband, four kids, two dogs, and three cats who need my attention. All four of my kids—now six, eight, ten, and fifteen—are involved in sports so the game and practice schedules are always on the to-do list. Some days the four kids are at three places, counting school, day care, and Grandma's—and I have to pick them up.

I also volunteer in our community. I'm involved with the local law library board, the PTA, the Lions Club, a local breastfeeding coalition, and a women's booster club for high school athletics. I'm active in local politics as well, and I have a consulting gig for the Supreme Court of Ohio.

Our life is managed chaos, really. Luckily, my husband, Paul, pitches in. But I still have a meeting, an appointment, or some other obligation every hour of the day.

There's a famous quote, from playwright George Bernard Shaw, about wanting to be fully used up before you die, that the joy in life is to be used for a purpose. That's my motto and that's how I run my life. It's constantly go, go, go.

Yet until recently, something important was missing from the list, at least from my personal list: exercise. I wasn't always this crazed, and I used to be pretty good about taking care of my health. As a teenager, I had been active. Then I began law school and sat all day. When I started having kids, I didn't do much of anything, exercise-wise. My hiatus from exercise and, really, taking care of myself was a long one—from 1992 until 2003. Over those years, I put on 30 pounds.

One day at work I felt lethargic, and I knew the lack of exercise and the extra weight weren't helping. I began to wonder, "Who am I to think my body doesn't need exercise?" I started thinking about my own emotional health, about giving the kids a good example, and I knew, deep down, that I'd be better off if I exercised.

A woman where I work always volunteers to lead coworkers in an exercise class that covers Pilates, small weights, and a little cardio. So I decided to join them. We exercise two or three days a week.

I had joined Weight Watchers about the same time, in 2003, after one of my friends kindly suggested it to me. One day, my leader, Dee, was talking about how women take care of everyone but themselves and how they should pay more attention to their own needs. When she said, "Put yourself on the list," I felt as if she was talking to me personally.

> "One day, my leader, Dee, was talking about how women take care of everyone but themselves and how they should pay more attention to their own needs. When she said, 'Put yourself on the list,' I felt as if she was talking to me personally."

It was really my Aha! moment. I had felt slightly guilty about exercising after work, thinking I should have been at home. She gave me permission not to feel guilty. From that moment on, I realized that my health is not a part-time job.

At that point, my decision to exercise wasn't about weight loss as much as it was about protecting my mood and staying healthy. I had ignored that aspect of my life for too long.

Now, working out is part of my life. Besides the regular, after-work sessions, I began to meet a friend for a Saturday morning workout at the Y. We walk or jog on the treadmill for a half hour and catch up with each other's lives. I've lost 25 pounds. I have also learned a lot of ways to squeeze in extra exercise. Sometimes I ask my husband to drop me off a mile or two from the house, whether we are returning from dinner or a ball game, and I walk the rest of the way home. I always keep a fleece jacket, a rain jacket, various hats, and sunscreen in the car so I can get in an impromptu workout.

Whenever possible, I also get the kids involved. Sometimes we walk to our mall, which is about a mile and a half away. Or maybe some of the kids will get on bikes and I'll walk or jog really fast along with them. Someone may decide to Rollerblade. We're usually dragging along a dog or two. There are times when I'm sure we look like a circus, but I don't care. I'm committed to this—for me.

TAKE-AWAY: Take some personal time

If you want to succeed at losing weight and improving your health, you need to carve out time for yourself—time to exercise, to de-stress, or to simply enjoy some solitude.

Losing It for Sugar Face

Lisa, 48, New York, accounting systems administrator

His name is Gary Anthony, but I call him Sugar Face. He was born June 21, 2002, the first day of summer. I was actually in the room with my daughter, Mylisa, when she gave birth to him, my first and only grandson. Just holding him took me back to when she was born—and that inspired me.

I decided then and there to lose weight because I wanted to be around to ride bikes with him and play ball with him. I've always been just like a big kid: I teach Sunday school to junior high kids and I'm a Girl Scout leader. But even simple games with a grandkid seemed impossible, given the shape I was in at the time. I didn't have just a few pounds to lose. In the previous ten years, I had let myself get up to 337—I figured I had at least 150 pounds to lose.

Weight had always been a struggle for me, but in the ten years before my grandson was born, it really spiraled out of control. Life had just gotten in the way of sensible eating. Being a wife and a mother and working full time as an accounting systems administrator took their toll. At one point, I even went on strike and didn't cook. I loved junk food. Often I'd grab a bag of cookies for myself for dinner.

Even before Sugar Face was born, I have to admit that the extra weight had been getting in my way. In 2001, I went to an amusement park with the Girl Scouts over in Hershey, Pennsylvania, and got on a ride but had to get off because I was too heavy and the seat was too small. I just didn't fit. That was embarrassing.

About a year later, I went on a winter outing with a church group, and we were all going tubing down a ski slope. To get started, the men at the top of the hill had to give you and the tube a boost, a big push-off. When I was ready to go, the guy whose line I was in gave the guy running the other line a look. It said: "Here's another two-ton Tessie I have to push off." I remember his eyes rolling. I couldn't wait until it was over because of that look. It ruined my whole weekend.

For years, the extra weight had given me backaches, too. But the absolute worst part was that after Sugar Face came along, all those pounds made me feel like an old, overweight, gray-haired grandma, the kind who can't move very fast. Don't get me wrong: I love being a grandmother. I just didn't want to look like one. I remember that my own grandmother was older and out of shape and would never play much with me. I didn't want to be like that.

To tell you the truth, I was having a bit of a midlife crisis. Here I was, in my early forties and a grandmother! I actually thought to myself, "Well, I can't afford a red Corvette so maybe I can reshape what a grandmother looks like."

I am a woman of faith, and a woman I go to church with had been losing weight nicely. A few weeks after Sugar Face was born, I asked her what she was doing, and she said, "Well, I walk in the morning." I knew I needed to do something, and I asked whether I could walk with her. So we did that.

After a while, I asked her what else she did to lose weight, and she told me about Weight Watchers. We live in a complex here in Queens, and they have meetings, but they were in the evenings, at seven, when I am often still at work. So I found a meeting near where I work.

> "A woman I go to church with had been losing weight nicely. I asked her what she was doing, and she said, 'Well, I walk in the morning.' I knew I needed to do something, and I asked whether I could walk with her."

I told them at the meeting that my goal was to lose 150 pounds. They explained that you don't set goals that high. So I got realistic, set short-term goals, and lost slowly but surely. It took me two and a half years, but I reached my goal. I actually lost more than that—about 162 pounds, because my weight now is between 170 and 175. I'm tall, 5 feet 10 inches.

These days, I don't worry about amusement park rides or guys rolling their eyes on the ski slopes. Junk food is no longer in control;

I am. But I do still have to remind myself when I get on the bus that I can now fit in the middle seat.

In the fall of 2004, Mylisa and Sugar Face moved to Louisiana, and they want me to move down there. But I like the seasons in New York so I'm staying here, for now anyway. I get down there when I can and they come up. Last year, I had my grandson for part of the summer. It was a blast.

When he visits, we do whatever he wants to do. He's nearly six now. We take turns riding his scooter, and I don't have to worry about breaking it. I bought him a tent, and we set it up in the living room and on top of the bed. I could actually crawl in with him. We just sat there, looked out, and giggled. That's when it occurred to me: I've made my vision of how a grandmother should look and act come true. No red Corvette needed.

TAKE-AWAY: Find a walking buddy

If you start walking regularly with a friend or a neighbor whose company you enjoy, you'll be multitasking in a good way—by exercising and socializing at the same time.

A Big Thanks to Mom

Brenda, 40, Wisconsin, teacher

In August 2002, I had a staff meeting at the Catholic school where I teach third grade. All of my colleagues were sitting around on old, rickety metal folding chairs, and the pastor was giving a sort of mini-sermon, as he always did at the meetings. Suddenly, I got a terrible calf cramp. I'd had them before, and I usually just walked them off, but I didn't want to get up and attract attention to myself, so I tried to shift my weight to see whether I could make it go away. One minute I was sitting on the chair. The next minute, I heard this loud crack and I was lying on the floor. The chair had broken under my weight. I guess I shouldn't have been surprised. Although I didn't know exactly how much I weighed because I hadn't stepped on a scale in years, I knew I was way overweight, and that made it all the more embarrassing.

I wanted to cry. I wanted the earth to split in two and swallow me up. Instead, I went into the bathroom and called my mom. She's the person I always turn to when I need comforting, but there was another reason I felt an urgent need to talk to her. She had told me the night before that she was going to her first Weight Watchers meeting the next day. She had been trying to talk me into joining with her, but I kept putting her off. I guess I didn't believe I could really lose weight because it had never worked before. But in that moment, when I was lying on the floor in front of everyone, my attitude completely changed. I knew I had to do something about my weight. I dialed her number and said, "Don't leave without me. I'm coming with you to the meeting."

When we got there, I was extremely anxious, mostly because I was worried that the scale wouldn't go high enough. The one in the doctor's office stopped at 300, and I knew I weighed more than that. Still, when I got on the scale I was shocked. For the second time that day I wished I could just disappear. But the group leader was wonderful.

She said, "It's going to be okay. It's just a number, and it's going to go down. We're going to do this together." She was so kind and understanding. I could have cried with relief.

The first week I lost 11 pounds, which was really motivating. But the meeting leader said that typical weight loss is about 1 to 2 pounds a week. That scared me. I said to my mom, "It's going to take me three years to reach my goal!" But she wouldn't let me get discouraged. She said, "It doesn't matter if it takes three years. This is our lifestyle now. We're going to be eating this way forever because we're making a total lifestyle change."

From that very first meeting, my mom was my rock—the person who cheered me up when I got discouraged, kept me on track, and set a good example. For the first six months after I started to lose weight, I was afraid to eat in a restaurant or even at a friend's house because I worried that I would eat too much and blow it. But my mom said, "You need to live your life. You're not going to be able to maintain the weight loss if you can't live with the program." That helped me to relax and try to incorporate the diet into my lifestyle. I see now how important that is. I was never successful at losing weight before because I didn't develop habits that I could live with.

I love ice cream, for example, but I'd never really learned to control how much I ate. My mom and I would go to McDonald's for a small ice cream cone every Thursday night after our meeting. I loved the ritual, and it helped me to see that I could still have my favorite foods as long as I ate them in reasonable portions.

> "My mom and I would go to McDonald's for a small ice cream cone every Thursday night after our meeting. I loved the ritual, and it helped me to see that I could still have my favorite foods as long as I ate them in reasonable portions."

We had another ritual that really helped. We talked on the phone after supper every day. We'd share ideas and recipes and talk about what we did for exercise that day. I joined a gym after I lost 100 pounds, then I switched to the women-only health club that my mom belonged to. I discovered that I just love step aerobics classes, and I do them three times a week. I feel as if our talks helped to keep me honest and on track. There were a number of times when I gained a little weight and felt really down, as if I was failing. But my mom would say, "It's all right. You know where you went wrong. Tomorrow is a new day. You'll just get back on track tomorrow." Hearing those words helped me to calm down. And the best part was, she was right.

In June 2005 I reached my goal weight of 180. It was so awesome to get there. I honestly never thought I'd see that number again. My meeting leader made a beauty pageant sash for me, and my mom was right there next to me, smiling proudly through the whole meeting.

My mom and I have always been close, but sharing this experience gave us a bond we didn't have before. My mom has lost weight, too. We've gone through the same emotional ups and downs. She understands exactly how I feel, and I understand her. When I look back, I think that when that chair broke in the school meeting, it was divine intervention. God gave me the nudge I needed to go to Weight Watchers—and He gave me my mom to help me through the journey.

TAKE-AWAY: Make changes you can live with
Finding ways to eat healthfully at restaurants or friends' houses or to incorporate your favorite foods into your meal plans will help you to make lasting changes and slim down for good.

Controlling My Weight— and My Destiny

Charla Krupp, New York, award-winning journalist and author
of *How Not to Look Old*

I grew up in the suburbs of Chicago, eating all the wrong things. In my family, dinners were very meat and potatoes. Vegetables were on the table to erase the guilt, but since they came from the can or the freezer, no one ate them, and they were always dumped out after dinner. Not many of the healthy foods were very appealing so, naturally, we all ate too much of the lethal stuff: steak, corn, potatoes, and lots and lots of bread, bagels, muffins, cookies, and brownies. There were some takeout places not far from us, so sometimes dinner was fried chicken with gooey coleslaw or hot dogs and french fries—and, of course, deep-dish Chicago pizza wasn't hard to get. Chicago is a food town, and it's hard to deny yourself!

My family definitely has weight issues. I come from a very carbo-hydrate-heavy home and I admit it: I am a carb junkie, too. It's my only addiction. I don't do drugs or drink that much, but I need my cookies every day! Thankfully, I realized that I had to relearn how to eat before I wound up too overweight myself.

When I moved to New York after graduating from college and worked at *Mademoiselle*, a fashion magazine, I realized that I really did have to learn a whole new way of eating. I was very motivated to lose weight. There's nothing like working at a fashion magazine—having to look at models and equally gorgeous fashion and beauty editors all day long—to embarrass you into eating less, shopping for a new wardrobe, getting a new haircut and color, and generally reinventing yourself. I knew I had to learn how to balance so I started to exercise. It was easy because it was social, a way to see my friends. I took up running and did a lot of high-impact aerobics classes. Then I bought a treadmill and did workouts with a personal trainer who came to my apartment. Now I love Spinning and do it as often as I can.

But ten years later, there were still these 10 stubborn pounds that just wouldn't come off. I had moved on to *Glamour* magazine by then, and I saw that our publisher had lost a lot of weight after having a baby. I asked her, "Tell me, how did you do it? What's your secret?" She said, "Weight Watchers." I was so lucky that right across the street from my apartment was a Weight Watchers sign. I ran right up there and joined.

Immediately, I was impressed with how liberating the program was. So many of my friends were on fad diets where they tell you, "You've gotta eat this and this and this. . . ." Not for me. I'm the kind of person who doesn't like to be told what to do; I want to eat what I want to eat, when I want to eat it. I control my own destiny. Weight Watchers just fits into your lifestyle, whatever it is. I lost the weight and became a Lifetime Member. I'm 5 feet tall, and at my heaviest I was 133; now, I'm 103.

I decided to lose weight for a couple of reasons. First of all, I want to look great in my clothes. I want to be able to wear a bathing suit in my home in the Hamptons—without having cottage cheese thighs. When you're around the beach and the pool, you just can't cover up all the time. I love knowing that if I am entertaining for a weekend, and I throw caution to the wind and eat what everybody else is eating, on Monday morning I can just go back to writing down my **POINTS** and in two days I will lose the weight.

I am also married to a super-skinny man, Richard Zoglin, who has a runner's body from running every single day; he has never varied in his weight in all the years I've known him. The challenge is that he does not need to be watching his calories, so in our homes we have his and hers of almost every food: whole milk and skim milk; regular salad dressing and fat-free; regular Coke and Diet Coke; real ice cream

"Whenever I return home to Chicago, I know that I'll have to repent for a week afterward because where I come from, food is unfortunately equated with love and caring. I've realized through all this that there's only so much I can do."

and fat-free; regular mayo and the no-fat version. And when he eats his super-fattening oatmeal cookies in front of the TV, I have my Weight Watchers crunchy mint chocolate bar.

Another big motivation for me is that I do a lot of TV interviews as a style and beauty expert. It's true what they say: the camera does add 10 pounds. You have to look good because everyone is looking at you and judging you in a nanosecond. In this business, you can't be fat! So you really have to watch it; you just can't let yourself go.

Which isn't to say I am not occasionally tempted. When my mother makes her famous chocolate chip cookies, it's very tough. But I know what I can eat. I know the consequences. And I have my mother trained pretty well by now. When I come to visit, she knows I need certain foods—yogurt, skim milk, blueberries.

Thanks to my losing weight, I think I've become a really great influence on my family when I'm around them. I have two young nieces who are very accustomed to eating mac and cheese, pizza, and hot dogs as a steady diet. But when they're around me, we have salmon and steamed broccoli for dinner. And you know what? They like it!

Both my brother and my sister, later in life, found that they, too, had to completely change their eating and exercising habits. And they did. Now, they both watch what they eat, and they exercise like crazy.

Whenever I return home to Chicago, I know that I'll have to repent for a week afterward because where I come from, food is unfortunately equated with love and caring. Love is shown by making a brisket! I've realized through all this that there's only so much I can do. I cannot change other people. I can only control myself.

TAKE-AWAY: Keep his-and-hers versions of your favorite foods

If you're trying to slim down and your spouse isn't, stock up on regular and low-fat versions of milk, mayo, salad dressing, ice cream, soda, crackers, and cookies. This will allow you both to eat what you like without harming your weight-loss efforts.

Rethinking Old Family Habits

Sara, 38, Pennsylvania, provider relations agent for a health insurance company

I grew up in the 1960s as the second-youngest of six sisters. With that many older siblings, you really have to fight for what's yours, including dinner. When my mom put food down on the table, you had to be ready to dig in or else you were left with scraps. My dad sometimes tried to slow us down by asking about our day, but it was still pretty chaotic. Although all the excitement and noise were fun, I know I picked up some bad eating habits. It never occurred to me to try to eat slowly—I was so busy rushing to get my share that eating fast became second nature.

My sisters loved me, of course, but as they got older, they tried to find ways to get rid of me. I was their baby sister, and if they wanted to go outside and play with other kids their age, the easiest way was by telling me there was something good to eat in the kitchen. "I think Mom's got some cookies for you!" they'd say, and off I'd run.

My parents were great, but I think that the awareness of nutrition and good eating habits just wasn't there at the time. And as a stay-at-home mother of six, my mom was just too busy to make sure we ate right. She made a home-cooked dinner every night, which is more than I can say for myself—as a working mom, I don't always have time to cook—but I know she wasn't monitoring the quantities we ate. And how could she? I, for one, was eating way too much, and the food was pretty heavy. A common dinner was a big pot of spaghetti with a stack of sliced white bread and butter, or meatloaf and mashed potatoes with gravy and lima beans. It never occurred to me at the time, but, looking back, I realize I probably overate partly for comfort. My parents had too much going on to give me as much attention as I craved, so I turned to food instead.

Because of all these things, I got hooked on food at an early age. Food became a hobby for me. If I went into the kitchen to look for a cupcake and found only two left in the package, I'd eat one and hide the last one so I could have it all to myself, later. I was already chubby by kindergarten—my class picture proves it. I never got a chance to learn what it feels like to feel full or to understand that when you're not hungry anymore, you stop eating.

Twenty years later, I was doing almost the same sort of things, but now I weighed over 300 pounds. Because I now knew that hiding food wasn't a good habit, I figured out other ways to eat without people seeing me. My husband worked nights until recently, and when he was gone and the kids were asleep, I'd serve myself a big bowl of chocolate-peanut butter ice cream and eat it in bed. It was part of my quiet time and my reward for working hard.

"Now I look back at those bowls of ice cream I used to have as part of my quiet time, and I think how ridiculous that was, to believe that a huge bowl of calories would make me feel better!"

Even though I felt vaguely guilty about these habits, losing a considerable amount of weight seemed impossible, so I did nothing. I know my sisters were worried about my health, but I'd get them off my back by saying, "No, I'm fine. My husband loves me the way I am, so why should I lose weight?" I had two kids, a good full-time job, and a nice home in the suburbs near four of my five sisters. Life seemed pretty good, except for the fact that I just kept gaining and gaining and couldn't stop. I truly thought I'd be fat forever.

In September 2004, a picture of me in my bathing suit made me decide to take charge of my weight. I was absolutely shocked. It wasn't at all the way I pictured myself in my mind! I signed up for the very next Weight Watchers At Work meeting and immediately started to cut back on how much I ate. The biggest sign that I was headed in the right direction came about three days later: I felt hungry for what seemed like the first time ever. After a while, I started to actually enjoy the feeling and the sound of my stomach growling!

It took me a little more than a year and a half to lose 143 pounds. One thing that really helped was to take the emphasis off food in my life. Now I look back at those bowls of ice cream I used to have as part of my quiet time, and I think how ridiculous that was, to believe that a huge bowl of calories would make me feel better! Now when my kids are asleep and the house is quiet, I'll read a magazine instead or watch the Food Network and write down ideas for my husband since I don't cook much anymore—he does most of the cooking now. And if I really can't keep myself out of the kitchen, I make myself busy preparing my lunch for the next day.

We're not exactly your picture-perfect family. Unlike my mom, we only sit down for dinner together about twice a week, what with after-school sports and activities—and when we do, it's my husband who cooks. Other nights, for my two kids, I'll cook an easy, usually microwavable dinner after school and accent it with some vegetables and a salad. On those nights, after they're in bed, I'll make something easy like salad or turkey burgers for myself. But the important thing is, we can all eat as slowly as we want to, without worrying about not getting our share.

TAKE-AWAY: Eat slowly

If you eat too quickly, it's easy to overeat before you realize that you've had enough. But if you slow down—and maybe even put your fork down between bites—it will help you to become aware of how much you're actually putting in your mouth and will give your brain ample time to register fullness before you've overdone it.

Dealing with Family Tragedy

Audrey, 39, Georgia, credit bureau account specialist

My husband, Bernard, was healthy and working. One day, he noticed a mass on his back. It started to grow, and it ended up being huge. In August 2002, we found out the terrible news: he had Ewing's sarcoma, a rare kind of cancer. The doctors tried to remove it, but the surgery didn't work. They did another surgery. Then they noticed that the cancer had jumped onto his spine.

The cancer spread to his brain. For the next eleven months, I went to the hospital every day that he was there. He had maybe one or two of those months when he was able to come home. Then he always had to go back in for chemo or some other treatment.

Before the diagnosis, we had a wonderful life. When we found out the bad news, our son, Amon, was seven and our little girl, Ryli, was only eighteen months old. When I found out Bernard was terminal, it was like swallowing the biggest, most bitter pill you can imagine. I just prayed.

Bernard died on July 24, 2003—he was forty. It was so hard, even with all the support my family and friends gave me. I felt that I had to be strong for my children, but sometimes I would allow them to see me grieve. I had plenty of time off from work, too. But as the weeks went by, I knew I had to get on with my life.

I was a thirty-five-year-old widow with two young children, and it was a very tumultuous time. Although I'd been heavy pretty much my entire life, I wasn't really bothered by it. And I hadn't given it much thought, of course, during all those months I cared for Bernard.

When I went back to work, I took up walking with coworkers again at lunch, something we had done before. One day, they started talking about the new Weight Watchers At Work meetings that were planned. They needed twenty people to join for the work meetings to be a go. I noticed that many of the women were smaller than I was—I wore a size 20—yet they were talking about joining. Then it hit me. My kids needed a healthy parent. So I joined. It was October 2003, just three months after Bernard died. I weighed in at 263 pounds, and I am 5 feet 7 inches. My goal weight was 170.

I focused on that goal. Joining did not take my mind off the fact that I was grieving, but it helped me to have a focus in my life. I went to meetings at work, and I also used Weight Watchers Online. I have learned to eat everything in moderation, and I've learned to measure portions as I cook or before I eat. I don't make separate meals for the kids. If I make veggies and grilled chicken, they will eat that, too. If they want chicken fingers and fries once in a while, I will eat that, too, but only a sensible portion. Now, if I am going somewhere out of the norm—a new restaurant, a retirement party—I will plan ahead. Say I have a piece of cake at the party: I will go take a walk a half hour later to make up for it.

I kept up the walking at work. My good friend Cheryl and I help each other constantly. If there are big bagels in the break room, she'll ask, "Do we really want to eat that?" I'll ask her, "Did you drink your water today?" She had much less to lose than I did, and she wore a much smaller size to begin with. So as her clothes got too big, she handed them down to me as my size 20s became much too big for me.

"I don't make separate meals for the kids. If I make veggies and grilled chicken, they will eat that, too. If they want chicken fingers and fries once in a while, I will eat that, too, but only a sensible portion."

I had some rough weeks, and I went through some rough times, especially during the holidays, at weddings, and at parties. But I stayed focused. By December 2004, fourteen months later, I had gotten down to 170, a loss of 93 pounds. Since then, I have settled in at 175, and I'm comfortable there.

I am so proud of myself. After I lost the weight, we went to a family reunion. I hadn't seen my parents in nine months, and they hadn't seen me with the 93 pounds off. They live in Missouri, and we're in

Georgia. My own father walked right past me. I said, "Daddy, it's me!" My family always gives out awards—certificates, really—at the reunions. They give them to kids who got straight As or to the families who had babies since the last reunion. They gave me a certificate for losing weight.

My life has turned around in so many ways. After I lost the weight, and after many months of grieving, I decided I would try to date. Soon after that, I met Michael, a wonderful man who lives nearby and values family as much as I do. We got married in September 2007. Now my life is coming full circle. We got through the grieving, my children and I, and the kind of man I have prayed for—one who is close to family, including his siblings—came into my life.

Everyone is overwhelmed with joy about my weight loss and my getting married again. I like to think that I've gone from tragedy to triumph.

TAKE-AWAY: Spend half your lunch break walking

Besides reducing the amount of time you spend around food, taking a midday walk can help you burn calories, boost your energy, and manage stress in the middle of the day.

Making Myself a Priority

Joseph, 29, New York, retail clothing executive

My parents were born and raised in the Philippines. I was born there, too, and we came to the United States when I was four years old. My family is very reserved. There are definitely no public displays of affection. I can't remember the last time my parents hugged me.

I am the oldest of four. As the oldest, I was really held to a stricter, more traditional, old-country standard growing up—and still am. On top of getting straight As, there were all these other expectations. I would wake up early and make lunch for my two younger sisters and younger brother. I worked part time even as a kid. It's the whole older-child syndrome in an Asian family.

By the time I was ten, my parents decided to put me on a diet. I was chunky and I had to wear husky-size clothing. That was hard on me. It was also hard dealing with the way my parents tried to motivate me. I remember when I was in seventh grade, there was a blizzard and school was canceled. I was at home, eating popcorn and watching television. My father said, "Oh, my! Look how fat your legs are." He said that, I know, in hopes of getting me motivated to lose weight. But it didn't.

The only thing I got comfort from was food. It's hard when your parents don't say, "I love you" because they are reserved. Eating was my way of feeling good. I got fat on steak and rice, especially a lot of rice.

By high school, I was up to 260 pounds, and I am only 5 feet 4. I was fat but not so fat that I was made fun of. I played football and baseball; I was athletic and strong. If anyone called me fat, I would challenge them.

Then, in February 1996, they took our senior pictures. I remember seeing my graduation picture and being horrified and saying I couldn't look at myself. I was disgusted. I decided to lose weight not for health reasons, but for vanity.

I joined Weight Watchers for the first time in 1997. And over a few months' time, I lost weight. I kept off most of it for years, then in

September 2005 I decided I had to lose more weight. What prompted me was that a guy who worked under me was heavy and people would tell us we looked alike. They said we looked like the Oompa Loompas, those chubby characters in the film *Willy Wonka and the Chocolate Factory*.

I thought, "I cannot look like an Oompa Loompa!" I weighed in at 193 pounds and set my goal at 164. I made it in about seven months. After that, I lost even more.

My habits and my outlook on life have changed. I work out every day, seven days a week. I do three days of weights and twenty minutes or more of cardio every day. I alternate between running, the elliptical machine, and the stair climber.

> "My habits and my outlook on life have changed. I work out every day, seven days a week. I do three days of weights and twenty minutes or more of cardio every day. I alternate between running, the elliptical machine, and the stair climber."

Years ago, my mother asked me whether I loved myself, and I just broke down and cried. We had been sitting, watching television, and I was eating a bag of chips. Like my dad, my mom was trying to motivate me to lose weight. She was trying to say that I was not making myself a priority, that if I loved myself I would lose some weight. But it was the wrong approach.

If she asked me now whether I loved myself, I would definitely say yes. After I lost all the weight, my parents said they are happy for me because they know I am healthier.

My weight was never an issue for my partner. I've been with him for nine years. He's 5 feet 11 inches and 170 pounds. He is lean and a good-looking guy. But he really noticed when I lost the additional 41 pounds. He said, "Wow! I never noticed how big you were."

Weight control is never going to be easy for me. The difference is: I've accepted it this time. I understand it. It's part of my life. In the past, I'd think, "Okay, I'm on vacation. I can eat whatever I want." Now I know that's not true. That's not me and it's never going to be me.

But the effort is definitely worth it. Yesterday, I looked in the mirror and said to myself, "I've never looked better." I just wanted to say, "Woo-hoo!"

TAKE-AWAY: Practice self-love

If you act as if you love yourself—by cutting yourself slack for mistakes you make, by taking good care of your body, and by comforting yourself in healthy ways (that don't involve food!) when you feel down—the feeling will gradually come naturally.

A Healthy Legacy

Fran, 59, New York, retired accountant and bookkeeper

Not long ago, my grandkids, who are eight and six, were looking at a picture of me at my senior prom. "Grandma, is that really you?" they asked. "You look so different!" And I did. It's not just the bouffant hairdo or the light-blue satin dress I wore with the dyed-to-match shoes and handbag. It's my weight. I was 170-plus pounds when I graduated from high school. That's one of the last pictures of me as a fat girl—and that size-18 prom dress was the reason I decided to lose weight.

I'd been chubby all my life. My father was a bread maker, and breakfasts were always a loaf of Italian bread with butter—delicious, but not exactly diet-conscious. I also ate lots of pasta and cannoli as a kid and didn't exercise. I was a klutz, and in grammar school I was self-conscious about my body and refused to put on a swimsuit or gym clothes. I'm sure my teacher wondered how I could possibly have my period every week, but as long as she let me out of P.E. class, I didn't care.

> "From the time she was born, I fed my daughter healthy foods. Now she's a dietitian, and she's teaching her own kids how to make the right food choices, which makes me really happy."

By the time I was a senior in high school, I was worried that boys wouldn't like me because I was overweight. So I was thrilled when Jim, a great guy I had met when we both worked at a local supermarket, asked me to the prom. But I was fed up with having so few clothing options so, shortly after the prom, I decided to lose weight.

This was in 1967, and Weight Watchers was taking the neighborhood by storm. Everyone I knew was trying it, so I did, too. And it worked. I reached my goal weight of 142 pounds within five months—and have rarely weighed a pound or two more than that for the last forty years. I eat extremely healthy during the week—I never have dessert—then I let it go a little bit on the weekends. And I exercise every day.

Sticking with a healthy diet and exercise has become so much a part of who I am that it's automatic. I never really think about it. But I guess my approach has affected the people I love. From the time she was born, I fed my daughter healthy foods. Now she's a dietitian, and she's teaching her own kids how to make the right food choices, which makes me really happy. When I was growing up, my family always said, *"Mangia! Mangia! Eat more!"* I raised my daughter differently. I tried to show her the value of moderation. Now her message to her kids is about healthy choices.

A while back, my grandkids were going roller-skating, and I went with them. They loved it, and I did, too. They have such an active grandma—it's no wonder they were so surprised when they saw that old picture of me. The girl in the size-18 dress, the one who hated to exercise, is long gone. The only thing left from that photo is my prom date. Jim and I have been married for thirty-eight years. He has loved me, literally, through thick and thin.

TAKE-AWAY: Aim for consistency

If you maintain healthy eating habits consistently during the week, you can splurge occasionally on the weekends and still lose weight.

From Single Mom to Diva

Kathy, 34, Texas, singer and purchasing assistant for a utility company

Ever since I was thirteen, I've been singing in churches, competitions, weddings, banquets, parties, bar mitzvahs, funerals. You name it, I've sung at it. I do a little bit of everything, except gangsta rap and ghetto metal. I love gospel and Aretha Franklin and Patti LaBelle. I think my weight problem started when I had to choose between softball—I was a very active, athletic kid, and played fast-pitch softball for fifteen years—and music at college. I picked music, and that kind of stopped the activity part of my life.

I got married at nineteen, had my first daughter when I was twenty, and my second when I was twenty-three. When I was two months pregnant with my second baby, my husband left. I was terrified—I had two lives depending on me for everything, and I'd never lived on my own. I felt abandoned, rejected, humiliated. That was the beginning of the really bad weight gain. I was an unwilling single parent raising two kids and worrying about money, and I compensated for my loneliness and depression by eating. I ate a lot of fast food, whatever was quick and cheap. I wasn't thinking about what I put in my body.

For a good eight to ten years, I gained a lot of weight every year. I never got on a scale. I knew I was overweight, and I refused to step on a scale and see how bad it really was. My doctor would ask how much I weighed, and I'd say 270 or 275. I only went to see him when I was sick so he didn't really focus on my weight. The first time in years that I stepped on a scale was at Weight Watchers. It turned out I really weighed 309.

One day I just knew I had to do something. I was about to turn thirty and I suddenly felt old. I remembered being healthy and in shape, able to jog and play ball and go tubing. I missed that. I remembered what it felt like to be able to sit comfortably in a fold-out chair at a baseball game. Or to go tubing down the Guadalupe River and be able to hold my head up. Or to be able to help my daughter learn how to ride a bike. I felt handicapped because I couldn't do those things anymore. I knew there was something better, and I wanted my old active life back. I wanted to do more with my kids.

Another thing that convinced me was seeing people, in my church especially, who had started losing weight. I saw with my own eyes the weight coming off. It got me to thinking, "If they can do it, I can do it." When I put my mind to something, I do it. So I made up my mind to do a 180: I was never going to be heavy again. It was like taking medicine for a sickness—I was determined to fix it.

I changed my diet—mostly by choosing whole-wheat pasta instead of white, corn tortillas over flour ones, salsa rather than sour cream—and I don't stuff my face 'til I'm sick anymore. Now I really pay attention to what I put in my body. I also started to exercise again. I walk about an hour three to four times a week, hard walking—where I sweat, and my blood pumps. I started out pretty slow, doing two miles in forty-five minutes, and now I go four and a half miles in less than an hour. It's kind of a meditation for me. I get my headphones on, listen to some good Christian music. It's prayer time, time to myself.

> "I changed my diet—mostly by choosing whole-wheat pasta instead of white, corn tortillas over flour ones, salsa rather than sour cream—and I don't stuff my face 'til I'm sick anymore. Now I really pay attention to what I put in my body."

The significant moment was when I got my 100-pound certificate. I was down to 209 and thought, "I'm almost down to the 200 mark; I'm almost there!" I'd promised myself a new outfit when I hit that goal, and that kicked me over the hump. "You're going to finish this now," I told myself. "You've lost a hundred pounds. You've come too far."

I've lost 167 pounds. The fun part is, now I'm a size 6 to 8, and I can shop pretty much anywhere. There's a shop called 5–7–9 because those are the only sizes it sells. I went in and bought a T-shirt just so that I could say I shopped there. I used to hate to have my picture taken because I always had a double chin. My mouth looked tiny, my eyes were all squinty, swollen, and puffy. I would look at the pictures and cringe. Now the double chin is gone, you can see the bone structure in my face, and my eyes look better.

My kids are proud; they've both said how happy they are. My baby, she's ten, loves that she can wrap her arms completely around my waist—she could never do that before. I'm also physically able to do things I couldn't before, like going out dancing. I didn't have the energy to do that when I weighed 309 pounds, and I certainly didn't want to shake my jelly in front of anybody! I didn't move around the stage much when I was performing because I huffed and puffed so much.

My friends thought that maybe I had lost some gigs because of my weight. I was the first runner-up in a televised Houston-wide talent show in December 2004. A thin young man won. He did have a great voice, but some people said I should have won. For the music industry, it's got to be the whole package or they don't want you.

People treat you differently when they think you look good. Men never gave me the time of day when I was overweight. Now men ask for my phone number. I'm dealing with a whole different set of issues, from "couldn't get 'em to talk to me" to "they won't leave me alone."

As a singer, people looked at me as the jolly fat person who always had a happy attitude. Now I'm a diva—strong and confident, energetic and comfortable in any setting. And I dress the part. I love to wear bright colors and shoes like my yellow patent-leather heels. My older daughter is a tomboy and gets embarrassed. She'll say, "Mom, people are staring!" But she likes it, too.

TAKE-AWAY: Look for weight-loss role models
Take note of people who've lost weight and gained considerable energy and vitality—and ask them how they did it. Borrowing their strategies could help you to sustain your motivation when it begins to lag.

Think about How Your Family Can Help

To remind family members of your weight-loss goals, literally post a "closed" sign in the doorway of your kitchen. It will remind you that you are done eating for the day. What are some other ideas for gently reinforcing to others what you're trying to achieve?

_____

_____

_____

_____

_____

_____

_____

_____

_____

_____

_____

_____

_____

CHAPTER 3

Working Nine to Five

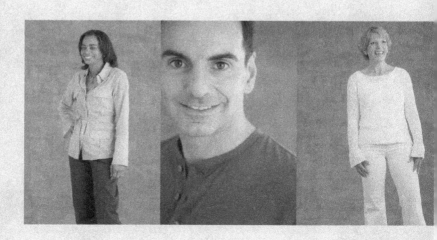

No matter how dedicated you are to your chosen profession, it's wise to consider how it affects your eating and exercise habits. After all, a variety of hidden challenges can sabotage your eating habits in any job. In the following stories, you'll read about people who faced on-the-job eating challenges, who needed to slim down to perform better in their jobs, and who grappled with maintaining both a career and control over their eating habits. By reading about how they handled their food and work issues, you'll be armed with insights to help yourself when you encounter similar work-related challenges.

Coming Clean with Myself

Sandra, 46, Pennsylvania, assistant vice president for a bank and a
Weight Watchers leader

I used to consider chocolate a food group. Chocolate candy, chocolate cookies, chocolate cake—I loved them all. I was naturally thin in my teenage years so I had the mentality that I didn't have to worry about what I ate. I'm 5 feet 8 inches and, for a while, I was 130 pounds, but I began to gain in my twenties because of poor eating habits, not exercising, and taking my weight for granted. When I had two children in my thirties, I used pregnancy as a carte blanche to eat as much as I wanted and whatever I wanted, especially fast food, fried foods, and sweets. I excused it as eating for two, and I gained 40-plus pounds with both pregnancies.

Then, as I became a wife, a mother, an employee, and a volunteer in the community, I didn't pay attention to what I was eating because I was so busy. I figured my weight would naturally stabilize, somewhere around 160, but then I'd gain another 10 or 20 pounds. Eventually, I went over that 200-pound mark that I swore I would never hit outside of pregnancy—then kept right on moving along. I knew I had to start bumping it down so I tried a few diet plans, but I didn't stay with any of them. I lost and gained 30 pounds various times. Finally, I decided that I had to get out of this cycle and get things under control.

In January 2004, I joined Weight Watchers when a coworker who was a Lifetime Member stopped by my desk and said, "Hey, I rejoined Weight Watchers yesterday, and you need to join next week." She'd seen me gain and lose and gain, and she'd listened to me lament about my size. At my high point, I weighed 215 pounds. Still, I was used to people telling me I looked fine. Deep down, I knew I needed to do this, but having someone else tell me I really had to join jolted me into seeing my reality. I decided that I had to stop playing this game with myself.

For a while, I was in denial. When we'd go out, I'd say, "This is a special occasion," and I'd justify eating whatever I wanted. For me, the hardest part of losing weight was adjusting to family celebrations and learning how to manage special events successfully. You want to fit into the situation but still be conscious of what you're eating. So I learned the importance of planning, of starting the meal with a big salad, and of stopping when I'd had enough instead of munching on chips or bread just because it was in front of me. I'm a fast eater, and it took a while for me to get used to eating until I'm comfortable but not full. I have to give my body time to catch up because if I eat until I'm full, thirty minutes later I feel terrible because I feel stuffed. I also started to get up and play volleyball with the kids at family barbecues so that I wouldn't eat to the point of distraction.

"In the past, one of my weaknesses was free food—eating the cakes, cookies, and doughnuts that were brought into the office. As I was losing weight, I would psych myself out of eating the free food by saying things like 'I don't know how long *that's* been out.'"

In the past, one of my weaknesses was free food—eating the cakes, cookies, and doughnuts that were brought into the office. As I was losing weight, I played these little mind games with myself: I would psych myself out of eating the free food by saying things like "I don't know how long *that's* been out; I'll bet it's stale" or "I don't know whose kitchen *that* came from," to take away the temptation. I also had this rule that if I really wanted to eat something that was against my goals, I had to go out and buy it and pay for it myself. Then I'd realize I didn't want it badly enough to do that, and I wouldn't have it.

I'm a very competitive person, and what really kept me going is, I wanted to beat that scale. I hated the feeling of facing that scale with a gain. So I'd say, "I'm not accepting any excuse—that thing is going down!" There's a famous quote: "Excuses are the nails used to build a house of failure"—and I really came to believe that. I set my goal to lose 2 pounds every week. That did not always happen—I had good and bad weeks—but my motivation became pumped up by the challenge of beating that scale. That mentality really helped me do what it took to reach my goal. It made it easier to say, "No, thank you."

I lost 70 pounds over twenty months, and I now weigh 145. I knew I was a lot thinner when my sister dragged me into a store to make me buy some clothes that fit. She gave me a size 6 that I swore would never fit, and guess what—it fit! I was like, "Wow!" I went from a size 18 to a 6. It's a wonderful feeling to set a high goal and to devote time, energy, and effort toward achieving it—then to finally make it.

TAKE-AWAY: Socializing isn't just about the food

By focusing on the social aspects of family barbecues, cocktail parties, and other get-togethers, you'll become more engaged in conversation and less caught up in mindlessly putting food in your mouth.

Losing Weight Surrounded by Food

Bonnie, 44, Maryland, studio manager for a commercial food photography company

It's not easy staying thin with my job. My husband and I own a food photography business so we're constantly around ridiculous amounts of beautiful food—incredible cheesecakes, lobster by the ton, Maryland crab cakes, chocolate chip cookies, every dessert imaginable! Being around food like that makes your mouth water, and I always had some of everything.

Really, though, my bad habits started before I even got into this business. Back when I was in my midtwenties, I was into body-building. I weighed between 135 and 140—I'm 5 feet 5 inches—and a lot of it was muscle. When I got pregnant with my son in 1991, I had been planning to do a state-level competition, but I had to drop out. I used pregnancy as an excuse to eat and I got as big as a house.

After that, it was one excuse after another—being a new mom, going back to work. Although I'd lose some weight, I always gained it back. When I joined my husband's company in 2002, I was probably around 155, so I was already chubby.

It just got worse from there. In the first year of my new job, I probably gained 10 or 15 pounds. We have food around us all day long. If we're shooting an ad for bread in our studio, we'll have an entire truckload of bread just to get a shot of one loaf! After the shoot, we pass it out to the crew, but there's only so much food you can give away, and we would end up taking tons home with us.

But the food we're shooting is the least of it. I'm in charge of craft services—the catering—and I have to order in breakfast, lunch, and snacks for the crew. I can't order diet food—the clients are paying a lot and expect all the bells and whistles—so in the morning there's always a table full of Danishes and other pastries, and for lunch it'll be pasta salad, chicken salad, or Maryland crab cakes. For snacks, there's always chips and salsa, and a basket of cookies, crackers, and candy. When I stopped for lunch, I filled my plate as full as I could. In between meals, I just nibbled all day long on all the snacks and the leftovers. I couldn't even tell you what or how much I ate because I didn't pay any attention.

Because of the weight I'd put on, it got so that it was hard for me to really do my job well. We have a back room with floor-to-ceiling shelves of props—it's like having a Pottery Barn or a Pier 1 right in our house. I spend a lot of time moving around on ladders, getting things, carrying bins, moving furniture. It's a very physical life, and when I was heavy it was very difficult because the spaces we were in are very packed and it was hard to maneuver around. I also got tired a lot, which is a problem when you're shooting all day long. I felt like I was carrying around a cinder block. It's also a very image-driven, age-sensitive environment—I'm surrounded by a lot of young, hip, cool people, and in comparison I felt old, dowdy, and unattractive.

Then in July 2003 we combined a shoot on Anguilla with a vacation with friends. When we got those pictures back, I couldn't believe what I saw. My friend is a size 0, and I looked like her fat mother! You don't gain 40 pounds overnight, but that's how it felt to me because it hadn't really registered before then how big I'd gotten. I was turning forty, and I said to myself, "If you don't do something now, you're just going to keep getting fatter and uglier."

I joined Weight Watchers the very next month, and I was amazed to learn that you can actually control your behavior around food. This is important for me because it's not always possible to control my environment. We will always have tons of food around us at work—I can't change that. But now instead of bringing home all the food from the shoot, I force myself to throw the leftovers out. I used to have the "people are starving across the world, so how can you throw food out?" mentality, but now I remind myself that my eating every last bite won't make the situation any better.

Our life is so crazy and irregular that I can barely plan anything—I can't tell you where I'll be from one week to the next. Working out is a disaster: I have a gym membership, but I go once a week at most because we travel so much. We live way out on a seven-acre farm in the country, have twenty-two dogs in our own kennel, and have to drive long distances to get anywhere. But I learned that in my daily routine there are plenty of ways to keep fit. When I carry the forty-four-pound bags of dog food, I do arm curls. Walking the trash bins down our half-mile-long driveway is exercise. Just getting to one side of our property from another is a workout if I choose to walk it instead of driving the lawnmower or the car.

> "I've learned that almost every restaurant will bring you a big plate of steamed broccoli if you ask, with a side of marinara sauce for dipping. That's definitely my fallback food for when I can't face another restaurant salad."

Around the studio, I did change a few things. Now I always order a big fruit salad along with the pastries for breakfast. The clients think it's for them, but it's definitely for me! I keep yogurt and water in the fridge and baby carrots everywhere, and I make sure to snack on them even if we don't break for lunch 'til three because if I get hungry and there's nothing else, I'll eat those Danishes. We still often get heavy pasta salads for lunch, but I make sure to have just a small portion. And every now and then we order sushi, which everyone loves.

When we travel, we might have to eat out five nights in a row, and it always seems to be at places that only serve wings and burgers. But I've learned that almost every restaurant will bring you a big plate of steamed broccoli if you ask, with a side of marinara sauce for dipping. That's definitely my fallback food for when I can't face another restaurant salad.

As long as I have this job I'll always be tempted to overeat, but now I know how to stay in control. It's so much easier for me to move quickly around the studio and have the energy it takes for a long day of shooting.

I used to have every size of clothes in my closet, but when I got down to 123 pounds I bought a pair of Levis and threw out all of my old clothes. They used to be my cushion because if I have stretchy pants around, I'll wear them. This summer I'll have kept the weight off for five years by taking responsibility for my own actions. Nobody else is going to do it for me. My motivation is remembering how it felt to be so big: invisible. Now I totally like that I fit in with the younger people at our shoots. I'm not the fat, middle-aged boss anymore.

TAKE-AWAY: Stay fit on the road

Don't let your travels thwart your weight-loss efforts. Walk around the city you're visiting, stay in hotels that have gyms, or bring an exercise DVD with you.

Acting My Way
to Weight Loss

Shuler, 40, New York, actor

In my work, I've often played gorillas and monsters because of my size, but I didn't want to look like either in real life. I am an actor for stage, television, and movies. I look kind of like a linebacker because I am a big guy, 6 feet 3 inches. My weight had always been reasonable—about 240 or 250—until about two years ago. One day in the summer of 2006, I weighed myself and was shocked to see that I weighed 289.

Before that, I'd never worried much about weight because I was active all through childhood and even into my thirties. My mom was the artistic director of the Georgia Ballet and my dad was an All-American football player, so I grew up playing sports, acting, and going to ballet class. In my first role onstage, I was Fritz in *The Nutcracker* at age five. In high school, I'd go to a ballet class in my football uniform, with mud still on it. I continued acting in musicals and plays through high school. I played high school football and college baseball for two years, then came up to New York to study opera.

I knew I had been gaining weight, of course, and I was beginning to notice it when I worked. I had started doing these shows that required me to run around and act like a gorilla. For instance, I did *Tarzan*, the Broadway musical, for a year. We were doing heavy gymnastics where we were flying on cables and stuff. Suddenly, I felt winded. I also noticed that when I was in motion and then stopped, part of my body, like my belly, kept moving. I had never noticed that until I started doing those kinds of physical stunts.

I think a combination of things made me gain. I was getting a bit lazy in terms of staying active physically. In years past, I would jog and that helped to keep my weight stable. It was easier to do that, though, before the kids came along. My wife, Paula, and I have a son, Grayson, who is four, and a daughter, Skyler, seven. When you have kids, you have to block out the time to exercise, and I really didn't know how to do that. I was eating the same amount but not doing anything close to the same amount of exercise that I used to.

Losing the weight wasn't about ego. It was about protecting my body and my health. Even at my heaviest I was still getting work as these big guys and monsters. I am usually a character actor, not the leading man type. Sometimes I am completely covered as a monster on stage, so I come out the door and no one knows who I am anyway.

But my excess weight just didn't feel healthy—it felt dangerous. I needed to be agile to do my job on stage, not to fall and get hurt. When doing these physical scenes, I would sometimes feel like my legs were giving out and my muscles would feel sore afterward. I also worried about twisting an ankle. I knew I needed to be at a weight where I could stretch easily and have good balance. In the upcoming play *Young Frankenstein*, I will play Frankenstein and I will be dancing. There is a scene where I will be doing a lot of falling. It's a very physical role so I need to be in top physical shape.

Something else that triggered my desire to lose weight was a photo. For one of the musicals I was in recently, everyone in the cast was supposed to bring in a baby picture and other pictures, as an ice-breaker, to get to know one another. One of mine was a picture my daughter took when she was about five. She was holding the camera, so it's angled up, and I look even bigger than I actually was. I had a big double chin and weighed nearly 300 pounds at the time. I was standing next to my wife, Paula—she's about 110 pounds and a yoga instructor—and it looked like my wife was at the zoo, petting the gorilla. It struck me that this is how my daughter probably sees me every day. And I didn't want that to be her image of me—at least, not in real life.

"In the past, I wasn't a conscious eater, and I became more of a conscious eater, figuring out whether I'm really hungry before I eat and cutting back on foods, such as desserts and breads, that I don't care about as much."

My manager and his wife had lost quite a bit of weight on Weight Watchers, and so had my publicist. I chose the Core Plan®, in which you pick and choose from a long list of foods and eat until you are comfortable but not stuffed. Just because of the nature of what I do and the amount of time I spend in the theater—sometimes it's ten, twelve hours a day—it's nice to know what I can eat without counting *POINTS*.

I also started to work out at a gym across the street from my daughter's school. I would take her to school in my workout clothes and go directly to the gym and do cardio on the elliptical trainer.

My starting weight was 289 in August 2006. By the middle of March 2007, I had lost 30 pounds. I'm now at my initial goal of 259 and trying to lose up to 10 more pounds. These days, I can really stretch without my belly getting in the way. I can touch my toes. My balance is better. I have more control over my body, which is necessary if you have to squat and run and fly on cables and do the other physical moves that are required in many of my roles.

The combination of watching portions and exercising is what really helped me to lose the weight. Now I look at going to the gym and doing cardio as part of my job. In the past, I wasn't a conscious eater, and I became more of a conscious eater, figuring out whether I'm really hungry before I eat and cutting back on foods, such as desserts and breads, that I don't care about as much.

I have also become assertive about what I need. The crafts table in show business—all those catered goodies on set so that we can take short eating breaks—is a horrible invention. They had a crafts table last week that had bagels, doughnuts, and brownies. I said, "Could we please get a bowl of apples?" By the end of the day, we had apples.

TAKE-AWAY: Schedule exercise as if it were a business appointment

When life is busy, you need to block out time to exercise. By scheduling your workouts in your day-planner and treating them as sacred appointments with yourself, you'll increase your odds of getting physical and staying that way in the long run.

Living through Downsizing—
in More Ways than One

Margaret, 39, California, marketing and sales manager

The dot-com bust made me start pigging out. I had been working in the San Francisco Bay Area, doing marketing for a company that provided media relations for small biotech firms. In September 2004 the company folded, leaving me unemployed, doubting myself, and feeling like a failure. For a while, I decided to try to work from home and do freelance PR, which involved a lot of cold calling and pitching my clients' stories, but this meant that I could eat whatever was in the house, whenever I wanted.

After about four months, I got another job similar to my previous one, but that one went belly-up, too. So I was back to sitting around at home, feeling bad about myself and basically eating my way through every day, trying to make myself feel better.

Without really realizing it, I'd put on about 25 pounds in six months—I'm only 5 feet 1 inch. But I was in denial about how much I'd gained. I just never saw myself as overweight, and since I never stepped on a scale, I was able to avoid facing the facts. Which meant I had no motivation to give up my new unhealthy habits.

My schedule went more or less like this: I'd sleep late, then skip breakfast. I'd have coffee, a big lunch, then snack all afternoon on candy, chips, whatever was around. If it was in front of me, I'd eat it. At dinner I got into the habit of having what I now think of as a party in my bed. I'd snuggle up in bed with pizza, chips, ice cream—not necessarily in big quantities, but more than was good for me. It felt safe in there, and because I wasn't eating at the table, I could fool myself into believing that it didn't count.

At home, it was easy to live in my stretch pants and sweats, but I was in for a shock when I started interviewing again and had to get out there and shop for real clothes. I remember spending a frustrating day in a department store trying on suits in the petite department. I kept trying outfits in the largest size they had—a 14—and they were all too tight. It was humiliating. I had to have a salesclerk go hunt something down for me. I remember feeling uncomfortable and depressed, but I still wouldn't accept the obvious answer—I had to lose weight.

There were other signs that I ignored, too. I was exhausted all day, I was overheated, and my feet and my back hurt. One of the things no one tells you about gaining weight is that your feet go up a size. So when I did finally get another job and went back to work in an office, I had to wear open-toed shoes because they were the only ones in my closet that fit.

Then two things happened to make me face what I was doing. My thirty-eight-year-old brother died suddenly of a heart attack. My brother going before my parents— that was scary! It made me think, If that can happen to him, am I next? And I wasn't helping the situation by taking such bad care of myself. A few months later I went to the doctor and found out that I had high cholesterol and high blood pressure. Now I was really scared. "You're smarter than this," I told myself. "You have to do something."

"I scheduled time to read labels and pick out a week's worth of healthy foods, so that I would no longer run out of food and have to grab something at random. If I lose that focus, I know my eating problems will come back."

The way I lost weight was by thinking about it as a second job and considering the people at Weight Watchers my boss. I put in time and effort and organized it like a work project. I would weigh the pros and cons of attending any event where I knew there would be food. I'd ask, "Is it really necessary for me to go or should I take a walk instead?" I scheduled time to read labels and pick out a week's worth of healthy foods, so that I would no longer run out of food and have to grab something at random. This sounds selfish, but I made it all about me, and I still do, because if I lose that focus, I know my eating problems will come back.

After my first meeting, I went out and bought a pair of walking shoes. I live in the city and don't have a car, but I used to take buses and cabs everywhere, even just a few blocks. I started walking to work, which actually took less time than the bus did, and after work I'd walk around the neighborhood before going home. If someone can't find me at lunch, they know I'm walking. I don't care if it's raining sideways, I'll be out there walking.

The walking helped me to lose more than 39 pounds, and the physical side effects are wonderful. My back and my feet no longer hurt. I have more energy and stamina. I sleep better. But just as important, it makes me more mentally alert. At work I can concentrate better and multitask. The old me would have been exhausted in the afternoon, but now, after a lunchtime walk, I'm totally wound up and energetic. And the walking helps me to eat healthier because after putting in all that effort, the last thing I want to do is blow it. I started to think about eating as a way to fuel my body, and I began eating more fruits and vegetables. In the process, my tastes changed—I'd never have believed that a piece of fruit would taste better than a piece of chocolate! But that's true for me now. And I only eat at the table—not in bed, not out of the fridge, not even standing up—so that I'm aware of every bite I take.

Getting my body back is my greatest accomplishment. I'm no longer worried that I'll be the next one to die after my brother. I'm doing everything I possibly can to be a healthy me—and the future's not scary anymore.

TAKE-AWAY: Eat only at a table
It's a mistake to munch in bed, on the couch, in the car, or straight from the fridge because these eating episodes don't really register, which can set you up for overeating.

A World Traveler Carries
a Lighter Load

Jan, 70, New Jersey, retired travel writer

I've always liked traveling—I've been to more than forty countries and six of the seven continents. Some aspects of traveling are definitely a challenge. When you're staying in someone's home or a simple hotel in a poor area, you don't have any choices—you eat what's set in front of you. But I love going places and seeing and trying different things. I really changed the focus of my travel since my husband died of pancreatic cancer three years ago. I joined a volunteer program and have worked in Mexico and Ghana, teaching English, and I am going to southern Italy next. Volunteering, it turns out, is a very different experience from traveling for work or leisure.

The Ghana trip in particular was a very intense, exhilarating experience. I lived in a small village where running water was almost unheard of and electricity was for the lucky few, but I was impressed by what wonderful lives the villagers had made without what we Westerners consider necessities. They enjoy their families and friends, and they have a strong moral code that comes from their churches; there was no crime in my village. My job was to teach sixth-graders, who, I quickly found out, are just as lively as sixth-graders the world over. They're so smart and energetic. They gave me, the "substitute," a hard time, but I learned that they could be extremely attentive when I found a subject that really interested them. From what kind of food is served on airplanes to whether American women have to cut off their hair when their husbands die—I wear mine very short—I spent a lot of time answering questions.

I was lucky: I lived in a guesthouse that was luxurious by Ghanian standards. We had air conditioning, electricity, and a formally trained cook named Florence. That was where the problem came in. Twice a day, Florence would serve me a huge piece of meat, a small bit of vegetables in sauce, and a big scoop of carbs. I ate more rice, fried potatoes, yams, plantains, and pasta than I'd had in years! Breakfast was always eggs and toast. Not surprisingly, I came back five pounds heavier, but as soon as I switched back to my lighter diet, they came right off.

I knew what to do to get those pounds off because I had joined Weight Watchers in August 2004, three weeks after my husband passed away. While he was sick, I realized that all the things I suffered from—high cholesterol, high blood pressure, and diabetes, things I took handfuls of pills for every day—were a result of my excess weight. I remember walking outside one day while he was sick and thinking, "If I don't do something, I'm going to go the same way." But I still had a chance.

What helped me to succeed was making my passions—traveling and cooking—work for me. At first, it seemed that the fact that I'm an ethnic-food junkie was going to be a real problem. One meal in a Mexican or Indian restaurant can blow my week. So I learned to cook all of my favorite ethnic foods at home, my way. I can do a mean Mexican meal with fat-free refried beans, low-calorie tortillas, a chicken breast, tomatoes, and fat-free sour cream and cheese. Moroccan is one of my favorite cuisines—I made a wonderful, healthy couscous salad the other day with dried cranberries, peppers, lemon juice, and spices.

"I learned to cook all my favorite ethnic foods at home, my way. I can do a mean Mexican meal with fat-free refried beans, low-calorie tortillas, a chicken breast, tomatoes, and fat-free sour cream and cheese."

I also decided that a sixty-seven-year-old can get fit, too. So I increased my lap swimming and began exercise classes for seniors, line-dancing, and going on long walks with my dogs.

For the most part, life is much easier now that I'm thin. I feel lighter, both physically and mentally. When I travel I can walk everywhere, even when our hotel is on the top of a steep hill, as it was in Mexico. In Ghana we did some long, hard walks, and it was not a problem at all. No longer do I walk into a room and think, "I'm the fattest person here." Instead, when I walk by a shop window, I look at my reflection and marvel.

The most important lesson I've learned is that it's never too late. For older people, it can seem much harder to lose the weight. Health problems and medications can encourage weight gain. We are more sedentary. Excess weight seems at first to be less important because, since we're in our older years, we aren't perceived to have the need to feel attractive. Well, guess what? We still care about how we look! And we don't have to feel like our age! If I hadn't lost the weight, I'd still be seventy this year, but I'd be fatter, my health problems would be worse, and I'd have a lot fewer years to look forward to.

TAKE-AWAY: Learn to cook ethnic favorites your way

These days, a variety of cookbooks can help you learn how to prepare low-fat, healthier versions of your favorite dishes from nearly every culture's cuisine.

Watching What You Eat
on the Road

Tom McCarthy, 39, New Jersey, radio broadcaster for the New York Mets

I've been working as a radio and television baseball announcer since I was twenty-six. I love what I do for a living, but in this job, I travel with the team, and I'm on the road a lot—about 110 days a year. One drawback is that I miss a lot of my kids' functions, like my boys' baseball games. It hurts when they struggle and I'm three thousand miles away. Luckily, my wife is unbelievable and always there for the kids.

The other drawback was even harder to deal with. Because I travel so much, my eating habits really suffered. I've battled my weight since I was a kid. I got into the habit of eating large quantities of fast food, and after high school I stopped doing sports and became fairly physically inactive. Then when I was traveling with the Trenton Thunder—then the double-A affiliate of the Boston Red Sox—I got up over the 300 mark; that was in 1997.

My lifestyle was not healthy. If I ate breakfast at all, it was an omelet at the hotel or an egg sandwich at a fast-food place. I ate most of my meals at fast-food places or at the concession stands or the media room at the ballpark. Even though I spent every night that I wasn't traveling at home with my wife and four kids, the bad habits I picked up the rest of the time carried over. Eating junk food on the run became addictive to me. I'd always been a disciplined person with my career, family, and money, but I'd lost control of my eating habits.

I didn't like the way I'd become—how run-down, sloppy, and old I felt. It was always on my mind. The main thing was that I was on TV, and even though I'd be on for only a minute or two per game, I thought it was unprofessional of me to be so heavy. I worried that if I ever lost a job because of my appearance, the guilt would tear me up inside. Still, it wasn't enough for me to change my habits.

In 2001, I finally reached my goal of being a major league broadcaster, doing play-by-play for the Philadelphia Phillies. Then in January 2005 I went for a routine physical to the same general practitioner I'd been seeing since I was five years old. This time, after he checked my chart, he looked at me and asked, "Tom, what're you doing?" I said, "Oh, I'm working for the Phillies now—" and he said, "No, I mean, what are you doing with your weight? You're only thirty-seven years old, you have four young kids; this is the point of no return for you." He made me feel like I was going to be dead before I was fifty—and it scared the hell out of me! He suggested gastric bypass, but I didn't like the idea of changing the inner workings of my body to solve a problem. I thought about it for almost two months and finally convinced myself that I had to make drastic changes to my life and that there would be no looking back.

I decided that I needed to learn to eat right while living on the road, with the options that are available. So I went to my first Weight Watchers meeting, at home in New Jersey. And I developed a routine: wherever we traveled, I'd go off and find a meeting. As soon as I checked into my hotel, in San Francisco or Atlanta or Houston, I'd walk to the closest grocery store and bring home cereal, milk, and fruit for breakfast. If I had to eat at the ballpark, I'd have a plain chicken sandwich, and I can tell you which ballparks have the best food and the worst. After I lost some weight and the arthritis I'd gotten from being so heavy got better, I started to work out in the hotel gyms, and now I do about an hour and a half on the elliptical when I'm on the road, and at home I walk and play basketball.

"After I lost some weight and the arthritis I'd gotten from being so heavy got better, I started to work out in the hotel gyms, and now I do about an hour and a half on the elliptical when I'm on the road."

I lost 137 pounds in about a year. I didn't tell people about it at first, but slowly they started to notice and keep tabs on me. Everyone in the Phillies organization was so supportive, and my wife was really happy, of course. My health had started to take a toll on her because she was afraid of my dropping dead one day, and she didn't know how to approach me about it. I know my kids will have their battles to fight in life, but I want them to know that this is one that they can win. I'm really proud of my oldest son, who's twelve. He's like my twin—exactly like me at that age, except that he doesn't have a weight problem. I tell him he's got to figure out for himself what is right and wrong for his body, so he watches the junk food and is active all the time, playing sports and running. Right now he's training for a 5K with my wife!

When I interviewed for my current job with the New York Mets in December 2005, I wore a suit that had been hanging in my closet since 1994; not only did it fit me, it was actually back in style again! I remember walking down the hall there and passing people I'd worked with in the past—and them not even recognizing me. Today it's such a relief not having the weight problem hanging over my head. I said to my wife the other day that I know it will always be a battle, but that's okay—it's worth it. Now when I go on the air, I don't have to feel embarrassed. I like that people are concerned with the content I provide, not with my looks. These days all that I worry about is the shiny spot where I'm losing my hair. Oh, and I still don't like the makeup thing, but I guess no men do, right?

TAKE-AWAY: Buy the fixings for healthy breakfasts and snacks while traveling

Even if you're staying in a hotel, head to the nearest grocery store and stock up on whole-grain cereal, skim milk, and fruit to ensure that you can have healthy breakfasts and snacks in your room.

Nursing My Portions

Barbara, 60, Florida, nurse

It's hard to be an obese nurse. For one thing, you're on your feet all the time, and that's difficult and sometimes painful when you're carrying a lot of weight. But there's also the emotional aspect. I've been a nurse for forty years, and patients sometimes looked surprised when they first saw me.

Every once in a while I'd hear a patient say something like, "Look at that fat nurse." It hurt. I felt ashamed and embarrassed. If you work in health care, people expect you to be healthy, and I wasn't. I had high cholesterol and weighed 252 pounds at my heaviest. To be honest, sometimes it was a bit uncomfortable talking to patients about their health when I clearly wasn't healthy myself.

When I got married in 1968, I weighed 150 pounds, but I gained weight with all three of my pregnancies and I never really lost it. I didn't exercise, and I ate way too many high-calorie foods. I loved ice cream, pies, cakes, cookies, doughnuts, pasta, sandwiches, french fries, and potato chips—and I didn't try to control my eating habits. I ate what I wanted.

Finally, I got tired of being heavy so in 2004 I started to cut back on what I was eating. I lost 20 pounds, but then I got stuck; I couldn't lose more. When my daughter wanted to lose weight and asked me to go to Weight Watchers with her in June 2005, I said yes since I wasn't getting anywhere on my own.

When I tried to lose weight in the past, I always thought about the 80 to 100 pounds I had to lose and the months and months it was going to take. That made me feel like there was no way I could do it. It made me feel hopeless. In one of my early Weight Watchers meetings, the leader talked about how futile it is to look at the long-range picture, and she said something that has stuck with me to this day. She said, "Just for today I can do this." That idea was very powerful for me, and I've probably said that to myself a thousand times since then. I don't think about the next day, let alone the next month. I just focus on getting through the day, and it really helps me to feel more in control.

While I was losing weight, I wrote down everything I ate every day. It made me more accountable. When I started to add things up, I realized there was a very simple reason I was heavy: I ate way too much of everything. I had an Aha! moment when I measured out what a half-cup of macaroni and cheese actually looks like. It's so much smaller than you think it is. Macaroni and cheese is one of my favorites, and I used to have half a plateful or more. That's three or four servings!

Working in a doctor's office, I'm exposed to a multitude of high-calorie foods all the time. Reps from drug companies, oxygen companies, home-health agencies, and other industries are always bringing us treats like doughnuts, cakes, pies, and candy. It's not easy to have that kind of food around constantly, and when I first started losing weight, the temptation was terrible. But I played a game with myself and the other girls in the office. I'd tell them to eat a bite for me. That helped me to stay straight. It was basically like telling them, "I'm not going to have any." Once I'd said that, I felt as if I really needed to stick to it because they'd all know if I failed. Their awareness helped me to stay strong.

Joining Weight Watchers was the best decision I could have made. The doctor I work for seemed to think so, too. He's an internist—and a stickler for healthy lifestyle habits. He didn't ever say anything to me, but I knew he thought I should lose weight, and I knew he was pleased when I did. After I lost about 30 or 40 pounds, he asked me whether I'd be willing to counsel overweight patients about losing weight. I felt really honored—and surprised. I'd certainly never thought of myself as a weight-loss role model before. But it actually helped me with my

"In one of my early Weight Watchers meetings, the leader talked about how futile it is to look at the long-range picture, and she said something that has stuck with me to this day. She said, 'Just for today I can do this.' That idea was very powerful for me."

weight loss, too, because I would try to practice what I preached.

I've lost a total of 82 pounds, and I've been able to stay at my goal weight—150 pounds—for more than a year. I've also brought down my cholesterol. Patients don't look at me funny anymore. I'm no longer just a nurse. Now I'm a healthy role model—not just for patients but for my kids and grandkids, too. And I love it.

TAKE-AWAY: Focus on daily goals

If you get in the habit of planning what you're going to eat and drink for today and you do this every day, you'll feel more in control and will develop a healthier lifestyle before you know it.

Stash Healthy Snacks in the Right Places

If you typically hanker for a snack while driving to the office or working at your desk, keep healthy choices within arm's reach. Then, once you reach your destination or have a moment for a break, you needn't go out of your way in search of something healthy. What else can you do on the job to keep the healthy theme going?

_____

_____

_____

_____

_____

_____

_____

_____

_____

_____

_____

_____

CHAPTER 4

Changing My Relationship with Food

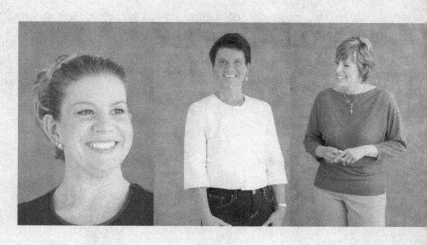

When life gets tough or you feel lonely, sad, or empty inside, food can easily become your best friend. Unfortunately, though, if you develop a habit of eating for emotional reasons, this can cause the number on the scale to rise. The men and the women featured in this chapter had a history of eating to quell uncomfortable feelings. As they recount the circumstances and painful emotions that caused them to turn to food for solace, you'll discover how they learned to manage upsetting feelings without using food as a crutch. After reading about their secrets to kicking the emotional eating habit and slimming down, you'll be inspired to follow in their footsteps.

Finding Me Again

Stacey, 40, Tennessee, fifth-grade teacher

When my children were young, I started to take Spinning classes with a friend at a tiny gym that opened up in Vermont. Three days a week at 5:30 in the morning, I'd go in my giant T-shirts and baggy sweatpants, and at first, sitting in the back, I could barely get through a class. At my heaviest, I was 180 pounds, and I'm 5 feet 2 inches. But I just loved Spinning. I feel it in my body, almost chemically; it's a stress reliever for me.

Then our instructor on Wednesdays stopped showing up, and the women in the class said they wanted me to teach. I said, "I can't teach a fitness class. Look at me!" I had this perception that because I didn't look like a fitness instructor, I couldn't do it. But I've been a teacher my entire life—I've been a lifeguard, a swimming instructor, a schoolteacher, and a mom—so it was a natural progression. And they really wanted me to do it. So I went to the director of the gym, who is a former Miss Universe, and told her the women in the class really wanted me to teach the class. She laughed at me and said, "Good luck!"

It broke my heart, I'm telling you. As I walked to my car, I thought, "Of course, I can't do that." But I remember putting the key in the ignition and thinking, "You know what? I'm going to prove her wrong. I'm not going to let that stop me."

What she said really hit a chord, though. My weight struggles actually started after I got married in 1990. I'm an emotional eater and the daughter of an alcoholic, and I think food was something I was trying to fill a hole with. I was using food as a replacement for a healthy relationship with my father and for intimacy. My self-esteem was suffering, and I had committed to an unhappy marriage and tried my best to make it work. I think I was eating to numb myself and not really look at what the problem was.

Over the years, I'd tell friends and family that I was unhappy about carrying this extra weight, and they'd tell me I was beautiful the way I was. Then when an old friend who was visiting town saw me, he said, "Oh, Stacey, you must be so unhappy that you've gained all this weight." I couldn't believe he'd said that to me—it was so mean. But it woke me up. It made me realize just how unhappy I was. My weight bothered me every day, but I wasn't doing anything about it. I hadn't looked at myself from the neck down naked for years. I was hiding myself—under the fat, under stretch pants and large clothes. I had to find me again.

When I joined Weight Watchers, my husband joined with me. We both ended up doing a triathlon after we lost weight, and in many ways, it helped us break the unhealthy cycle we were in. But it didn't save our marriage. I knew I'd reached a turning point with my weight when I decided I was going to let go of my marriage and get divorced, that I would have the courage to do that.

> "I look better at forty than I did when I was thirty. I love my quads—my legs are strong and the cellulite's gone. Sure, I have stretch marks and crow's feet, but I feel beautiful on the outside because I let go of a lot of trash that was on the inside."

It was about getting out of an unhappy relationship and taking care of me—and not feeling guilty about it. That's not being selfish; that's self-preservation.

These days, I feel great. I have tons of energy. Looking back, I feel as if the comment by Miss Universe was a pivotal moment in my life. After that, I got my Spinning instructor's license, and I've been teaching it now for five years. I lost 26 pounds from Spinning and another 27 pounds through Weight Watchers.

I'm in Tennessee now, and I teach Spinning three days a week. People who take my class here met me when I weighed 125 pounds, not 180, and they can't believe it when I show them my old pictures. I look better at forty than I did when I was thirty. My body loves being a size 6, and I love my quads—my legs are strong and the cellulite's gone. Sure, I have stretch marks and crow's feet, but I feel beautiful on the outside because I let go of a lot of trash that was on the inside. When you take care of yourself and you let your light shine, you give other people permission to do that for themselves. That's a wonderful gift.

TAKE-AWAY: Speak kindly to yourself

Instead of telling yourself that you can't or won't achieve a goal that's important to you, bolster your resolve and your can-do spirit by giving yourself a pep talk and reminding yourself how strong and capable you really are.

Stopping Sneak Eating

Melissa, 48, Pennsylvania, court reporter

From the time I was a little girl, I was a sneaky eater. I can remember tiptoeing into the kitchen, gently opening the cupboard where my mom kept old mayonnaise jars full of cookies and crackers, slipping some out, and eating them as quickly as I could. I've always had a sweet tooth, and I craved foods that weren't good for me. Then when I was a teenager and became heavy, I got into the mind-set of, "It's not okay for me to eat this so I have to sneak it."

It just got worse as I grew up. I did lose weight after having my kids, but then in my early thirties the pounds came back—and I started to sneak food again. After coming home from work to an empty house, the first thing I'd reach for was potato chips. I'd eat them 'til I had enough, then have five or ten cookies, or else dig into the ice cream container with a spoon. When I heard the garage door opening, I'd throw the ice cream back in the freezer.

I'd do it when people were home, too. At night, when my husband was watching TV, I'd sneak into the kitchen and bring food into the family room or upstairs to the bedroom, and eat it alone. Sometimes I'd buy cookies on the way to work and eat them in the car, and if I baked a cake or brought home cookies "for my family"—which was always my excuse!—I'd end up eating almost all of them myself. No one ever knew what I was doing.

After I'd pig out like that, I'd ask myself, "Why, why, why do you do this to yourself?" But as soon as I started eating, the impulse took over and I couldn't stop. I was ashamed of my weight and my lack of control.

Boy, did I want to lose weight! But doing it on your own is so hard. I had actually lost a lot of weight ten years ago, mostly through exercise, but since I never faced my food addiction, it all crept back on.

Today, after I've lost 86 pounds, it's still tough, and sometimes I falter. Just last week I made a pan of brownies and ate them all, just because they were sitting there in the refrigerator.

For the most part, I've learned how to control the sneak-eating pattern because now I recognize what triggers it. Since it's really just certain foods that bring on the impulse—sweets, chips, basically anything unhealthy—I no longer have them in the house. These days, I stock my kitchen with healthy things like dried fruit, fresh fruit, yogurt, and high-fiber cereal. I can even eat alone now, as long as I stick to healthy foods, and when I get home from work and want to snack, I reach for something special but not dangerous, like dried plums with a cherry essence. For me, it's all about mind over matter.

> "For the most part, I've learned how to control the sneak-eating pattern because now I recognize what triggers it. Since it's really just certain foods that bring on the impulse, I no longer have them in the house."

I love feeling more in control around food. I also must admit that I love being treated differently now that I'm thin. This should bother me, but it doesn't. I like that people at work talk to me more now. I realized how much happier and nicer I am now because one day someone at work stopped and told me how happy he was for me and that my personality was so much more beautiful. That really took my breath away.

TAKE-AWAY: Give your kitchen a makeover

Get rid of junk foods and trigger foods—the ones you often overeat—and restock your kitchen with healthy items like fresh and dried fruits, whole-grain crackers, yogurt, and high-fiber cereal.

Weight and Relationships

Marie, 41, California, deputy director for a child support collection agency

I met my first husband at a dance club in 1995, and not long after that we were married. He was in the navy and had to leave town on six-month tours, so I knew he'd be gone a lot. What I didn't know was how that would affect me—and my eating habits.

I was alone all the time because most of my friends were single, and they'd go out dancing or to the bars at night. I didn't feel comfortable joining them because I was married, so I stayed home, watched TV—and ate. I'd eat anything that made me feel better—pizza, spaghetti, fast food. Since I was home alone, I kept going back for more and more. I could polish off a whole pizza by myself and still be hungry—or at least think I was. What I believe now is that I was hungry for interaction, for attention, for someone to be there with me. I wanted a husband who was home, but, more than that, I wanted to be with someone who liked to laugh, travel, share his emotions, and experience new things.

The marriage lasted seven years. When we got married, my weight was about 155—not bad for someone who is 5 feet 7 inches—and by the end I weighed over 200 pounds. I was miserable. I lost some weight because of the stress of the divorce, but then I started dating a guy who was totally inactive and a big eater. I put all the weight back on—and then some. Fortunately, that relationship didn't last long.

It was December 2002. I was single, fat, and unhappy. My weight gain, I realized, had paralleled my unsuccessful relationships, but now I was alone—and I decided it was time to try to get healthy and get my weight under control. I enrolled in Weight Watchers weighing 250 pounds, and I bought a treadmill and began to walk two miles every morning. I hadn't exercised in nearly ten years, and the first couple of days I thought, "Oh, my God, I can't do this." But I remembered someone telling me that if you do something for 30 days, it becomes a habit, so I decided to stick it out. It took more than 30 days—probably more like 130—but, eventually, exercise became a routine part of my morning. After a while, I didn't think about whether I was going to do it or not. I just did it.

After nine months, I began to increase my mileage and pace, and I added some aerobics classes to my routine. Finally, two years after I joined Weight Watchers, I reached my goal weight: 150 pounds. I felt so good to be slim and fit. I felt like me for the first time in years.

I had been dating off and on but hadn't met anyone who was right, so I put an ad on Match.com. I can't remember exactly what it said, but the gist was this: "I'm looking for someone who is active and likes to exercise and have fun." A man named Ray responded, and we went out for dinner. He was a triathlete and was totally motivated to stay fit. He was different from anyone I'd ever dated in other ways, too—funny, mature, interested in having kids, able to open up emotionally. We met in May 2005, and by October 2006 we were married.

Like my old relationships, my new marriage has an influence on my life—except this time the influence is healthy. Thanks to my husband, I've tried all sorts of things I never thought I would: karate, swimming, running, backpacking, bike riding, snowboarding. I exercise every day, and if I don't feel like it, he encourages me to do it. I've been a good influence on him, too. Because he's always been so active, he's never paid much attention to his diet. I introduced him to the idea of healthy eating, and now salads are a regular part of his day.

> "I hadn't exercised in nearly ten years. But I remembered someone telling me that if you do something for 30 days, it becomes a habit, so I decided to stick it out. After a while, I didn't think about whether I was going to do it or not. I just did it."

I'm proud of my size-4 body and my sculpted arms—you can actually see the muscle now—and I'm proud of my weight loss. But I'm most proud of my marriage. I finally realized what I was looking for in a relationship, and I found those things with Ray. For the first time ever, I can say that I'm in a truly healthy relationship, emotionally and physically.

TAKE-AWAY: Give new habits time to stick

Change doesn't happen overnight. When you're revamping your eating or exercise habits, it often takes six months for a new habit to feel natural or nearly automatic, so make a commitment to stick with it for at least that long.

Finding the Bubbly Girl Again

Sandy, 33, New York, high school Spanish teacher

As I gained weight, I started to lose my sense of me, who I really was on the inside. My husband always used to say that it wasn't my body he fell in love with. It was my bubbly personality—that's what attracted him to me. But by the time my weight hit its highest point, I could feel that bubbly part of myself slipping away. It was getting harder and harder to put a smile on my face.

The unhappier I was about my appearance, the more I avoided thinking about it. Instead, I would focus on my responsibilities as a mother, a wife, and a teacher and do things for everyone else except myself. I stopped taking care of myself and caring what I looked like—I kept my hair really short and I wore sweats a lot or whatever I could find to fit. It got to the point where I didn't really have a sense of who I, Sandy, was anymore.

Gradually, I started to worry about how my looks affected my family, especially my husband. I worried that he would be ashamed to be seen with me. Once I asked him whether he was sure he wanted me to come to his office party because I was convinced that I'd embarrass him. He said, "I love you for you and I'm not going anywhere." But I had this crazy fear of losing him. At times, I felt as if my mood was sliding into a depressed state.

And being that unhappy made me eat more, so I gained more. I knew that I felt down because of the weight gain, but it was easier to ignore than to figure out how to fix it.

When my daughter got older—she's seven now—she would make comments about my belly or she'd tell me I had a big butt. She wasn't being mean; she was just being truthful, the way kids are. They were just her observations that her mom was bigger than other moms. Which was true. But that made me step back and realize that my weight and what I was doing with food weren't affecting only my life but also the lives of my family.

Finally, in July 2004, my mother-in-law asked me what was going on because she could tell that something was bothering me. She told me that she noticed the life draining from me and said she wanted to help if she could. I confessed that my weight was upsetting me, and she said I could attend Weight Watchers with her if I wanted to. I did—and I'm glad I went.

I lost 95 pounds and I have kept them off, mostly by cutting my portions way back. I used to match my husband bite for bite, and he's a foot taller than me. I don't do that anymore.

> "I lost 95 pounds and I have kept them off, mostly by cutting my portions way back. I used to match my husband bite for bite, and he's a foot taller than me. I don't do that anymore."

But the most important change I made is on the inside. I have so much more confidence now that I know people are paying attention to me, not to my weight. I have never been this thin, not even as a teenager, and I'm more outgoing now because I feel good about myself. I don't care as much what other people think of me, and I've discovered how to have fun again.

At a Christmas party last year, I even got up and danced on the bar—and I was totally sober. I did it just because I felt like it, and I didn't mind if I was the center of attention. My husband couldn't believe it. I can't remember what song it was, but in my mind the jukebox was playing one of my favorites. That's when I knew that the old me—but a better version—was back.

TAKE-AWAY: **Don't match your dining companions bite for bite**
Rather than trying to keep up with how quickly or how much someone else is eating, it's better to focus on enjoying what you eat and consuming enough to satisfy—but not stuff—yourself.

Stopping the
Junk-Food Habit

Ann, 41, New York, high school history teacher and Weight Watchers leader

I used to dream about frosting—always German chocolate cake flavor, my favorite. For most of my life, I thought there was nothing like a can of frosting when you're stressed out. Open the top, get a spoon, and just eat. I'm not sure why it was so comforting, but it always was.

Other times I'd eat a whole pizza, a lot of french fries, or a cake when I was upset. I was a junk-food junkie. Deep down, I still am. But I've learned how to stop myself, and I took off 217 pounds in the process. When I started Weight Watchers on July 9, 2000, I weighed in at 358 pounds.

My story could have turned out a lot differently. About an hour before I joined Weight Watchers, I was in my doctor's office, asking for a referral to a bariatric specialist for gastric bypass surgery. My general physician said, "No, you are not a candidate." He thought that I would lose, at best, 50 pounds. And he reminded me that I needed to lose hundreds. I said, "Thanks for pointing out the blooming obvious."

It took me almost two years to reach my original goal of 167. I took off more in the next few months and finally settled in at 141 pounds. I am 5 feet 7 inches. I'm now a Weight Watchers meeting leader.

I still think about frosting—and sometimes I am tempted to go back to my old ways, eating a can of frosting to relieve stress. One night, my car was broken into while I was leading a meeting. The thief took my cell phone and my iPod. I was upset. All I wanted, I admit, was a can of frosting. Luckily, the market was closed.

I share with my members what helped me to become a recovering junk-food junkie, what helped me to make better food choices and lose the weight. It boils down to two things: being organized enough to plan ahead on food choices and being very good at talking positively to myself.

Soon after I joined Weight Watchers, I sat back and thought about why I had been successful in every other part of my life but not with weight control. I'm a very successful teacher, and I thought about why that was so. I concluded that it's because I plan ahead. I already know what I'm doing in third-period history class next week. When I plan a museum field trip, I organize everything ahead of time—the buses, the chaperones, where we'll have lunch, bathroom stops, all of that.

I figured that if I could apply this knack for planning ahead and organizing to my weight-loss plan, I might be more successful this time. So, every night, I would plan the next day's meals—all of them. I'd figure out that I was having oatmeal and a banana for breakfast, a salad with turkey and croutons for lunch, yogurt for a treat, and so on. If I hadn't done that, I would have been off the plan. By rigorously planning like this, I now make better food decisions. I still do this.

I also exercise a lot. I'm up every day at 4 a.m. and join a friend at the gym. Often I do forty-five minutes on the treadmill and then twenty minutes of weights or a forty-minute walk. Exercising relieves my stress, helps me to make better food decisions, and helps me to maintain my weight loss.

"More than once, I have also said to myself: 'If you eat that can of frosting, is it worth it?' Usually, of course, the answer is no."

The other tool that helps me with food decisions is my realistic, positive self-talk. When I'm tempted, I often say to myself, "My clothes will continue to fit if I don't overeat" or "I don't want to undo my progress." More than once, I have also said to myself, "If you eat that can of frosting, is it worth it?" Usually, of course, the answer is no.

Left to my own devices, I'd still be a junk-food junkie. I know it. I struggle every single day. Instead of giving in, I give myself a pep talk. Sometimes I distract myself when I hear the frosting calling. I do housework or call a friend. Mostly, I choose to stay away from junk foods, especially frosting, chocolate peanut butter cups, crackers, and peanut butter. I cannot eat certain foods because I know that once I start, I will just keep on eating them.

But sometimes, the extra **POINTS** are worth it. The diner in my neighborhood occasionally has these wonderful Polish potato pancakes flavored with parsley and onion. The next time they have them, I'm going to eat lettuce the rest of the day so that I can have a potato pancake. They're wonderful. The phrase I use all the time when making food decisions is: "Is it worth it?" Potato pancakes, once in a while. Frosting, no.

TAKE-AWAY: Distract yourself

When cravings for sweets or junk food threaten to derail your healthy eating plan, distract yourself by calling a friend, going for a walk, writing a letter or an e-mail, or doing something else that doesn't involve food. In all likelihood, the cravings will pass in a matter of minutes.

Learning to Love Me

Sarah, Duchess of York, author, philanthropist

I didn't always know I was an emotional eater. Before I began the Program, everything in my life revolved around food—I was always looking for my next fix. Whether I was happy or sad, or even tired. Actually, that is the perfect example. If I had been this tired a decade ago, I would have reached for the nearest bagel because I thought it would give me a kick. Now I know that when I'm tired, I need sleep, not food.

I'm now in the maintenance phase of my weight loss and will always track my *POINTS* values because that's how I maintain my weight. The sooner you see that you're losing control, the sooner you can pull yourself together. For example, now I use exercise as a way to pull myself together. One of my favorite experiences in the world is feeling fresh air on my face and hearing the wind in the trees. I hate to feel confined indoors, so even when I'm on the road I find a park to jog (slowly!) in. It's never boring—and I always prefer walking outside to working out in a gym on a treadmill. It's all about learning what your triggers are, then finding solutions to head them off.

I have my moments. Last night I had an extra glass of wine. But after my slipup, I do my best to get back on track the very next second. You know how the second hand on a clock always keeps moving? I've realized that so should you. Time doesn't stop for us. We can eat fifty-nine million boxes of caramel corn, and that second hand will keep ticking. The very next second is your chance to get back on track and ask yourself, "Why did I need that food?" Maybe you were upset because a man didn't call, for instance, or you felt lonely or isolated. That realization is an opportunity: you can suffocate yourself with food to cover the feeling, or you can embrace the feeling and move forward.

When I find myself overeating, I get up—literally—and walk away. Do something altogether different. I'm very strong on this point: you have to find a way to get around whatever you believe are your roadblocks, your excuses. For example, I met a woman who uses a wheelchair and takes steroids, and she said, "I'm never going to lose weight." But through the encouragement of her Weight Watchers leader and other members, she has lost 75 pounds and is walking for the first time in years!

My big excuse was I thought I was unlovable, unworthy. I remember the self-hatred vividly. I thought no program could ever "fix" me. I was sure that I would sabotage my success on WW. But I stuck with it. I needed to understand that the "fat lady"—that little voice in your brain that constantly criticizes your body—will never completely go away. You'll probably always look in the mirror and find a figure flaw—"I hate my backside" or "My thighs are too fat." That's just the fat lady talking! Over the years I've learned to talk to the fat lady and her committee. I say, "Thank you for coming, but I'll be okay. I'm going to win this one."

> "Understand that the 'fat lady'—that little voice in your brain that constantly criticizes your body—will never completely go away.

TAKE-AWAY: Silence your inner naysayer

When a little voice inside your head points out your flaws or tries to convince you that you won't achieve your goal, tell it to hush and remind yourself that you do have matters under control.

Feeling My Feelings, Not Stuffing Them

Ed, 38, Illinois, actor, Weight Watchers trainer and leader

For pretty much my whole life, I have gained and lost weight, gained and lost weight. In high school, college, and afterward, I'd gain until I sometimes reached 240, then diet and get down to 170 or so.

Now, I understand why: I'm an emotional eater. When I'm thrown by upsetting events, or when I don't want to deal with my feelings, I overeat, especially comfort foods or junk foods like jelly beans, cookies, cake, candy corn, or ice cream. Even as a kid, I did this.

By the third grade, I was already chubby. By the end of my sophomore year in high school, my weight hit 240. My younger sister and her friends made fun of me, nicknaming me "Bubba." That hurt.

That summer, before my junior year, my family was preparing to host a German exchange student. So I thought, "I'd better lose weight before he gets here, so he'll think I'm cool." I essentially starved myself and got down to 170. I didn't stay at that weight for long, though, and it was largely because of my emotional eating.

My mother died of cancer, back in 1993. She was only forty-seven. I was twenty-three and devastated. She was a doting mother, and we were close. After the funeral, friends came over to the house with food. There was a big plate of brownies, and I remember starting to eat them, a lot of them, and saying in my head, "What does it matter? Does it really matter if I weigh 170 or 240?" I was in pain, and I wanted to eat, not worry about my weight or deal with my grief. I ate probably three-quarters of the plate of brownies.

Within three months I had put on 30 pounds; once again, my weight was on its way back up. Besides using food to cope with feelings I didn't want to deal with, I think I was fearful of really being happy. Somewhere along the line, I got the idea that if you are not at an attractive weight, you are not entitled to certain experiences, including happiness. In the gay community, having a lean body is extremely important, and I felt that pressure. But the flip side of this twisted logic was that whenever I had lost weight and was at a good weight for me, I somehow thought I didn't deserve to be at that weight or to be happy.

By 2001, I slowly came to realize that my excess weight was messing up my life and my career. I was pursuing my acting dream, and still am, but with my weight problem I was most likely to be offered the fat guy character roles, and I wanted starring roles. So I got more serious about weight loss. I tried a high-protein diet and lost 15 pounds. But it was too restrictive. I was tired of eating meat all the time.

Looking for something I could stick with, I went to Weight Watchers in March 2002. I weighed in at 185. By May 2003, I was down to 153, my goal. For nearly the last five years, I have stayed at that weight, give or take a couple of pounds, and I'm now a Weight Watchers leader.

I've done well, but the fear that emotional eating will get the better of me again still lurks. That anxiety has lessened a lot, but it is still there sometimes because the transformation from yo-yo dieter to someone who maintains a healthy weight is a long process and it happens in stages. First your behavior must change, and then your sense of who you are must shift. You need to learn to think of yourself as a thin person, not as a fat person who happens to be thin right now.

I am not completely that new person yet, but I am getting closer. In fact, sometimes I astonish myself with my control over my eating habits. Like last Christmas, when I went to my aunt's in Massachusetts, where I grew up. For many people, including me, holidays are an emotional time, full of mixed feelings. The first thing my aunt did when I got there was take me on a tour of the house to show me where the goodies were. There was a candy dish with foil-wrapped dark chocolate bells on top of the piano, another dish with homemade candy in the living room, and a bowl of pink-and-white mints on top of the china cabinet. There were Heath Bar cookies on the kitchen counter. I remember looking at them and thinking, "Boy, those look good!" Then I told myself, "Ed, you can have one Heath Bar cookie per day"—and that is what I did, every day that I was there.

To maintain my goal weight, I've adopted many new habits. I've never been much of a cook and I'm still not. So I focus on eating "whole foods," which, to me, means a lot of salads and putting something simple in the oven, like a chicken breast. I've also found my inner athlete. I'm as surprised as anyone, but I now exercise five days a week. I do cardio and weights. I bicycle and go downhill and cross-country skiing when I can. I have become a runner.

I have finally realized that keeping the weight off comes down to my resolve to make both mental and behavioral changes. I have to remember that a crisis, big or small, has the potential to throw me into a fit of emotional eating, and I have to remember that I need to cope in other ways besides eating.

I am dating this guy right now who is also an actor. Jason could model for Abercrombie and Fitch. He's really in shape and looks great. My body is just average, even though I have been working with a trainer for months. The best I can say right now is that I have a runner's physique—slender but not pumped up.

"The lightbulb went on: whether I ate or didn't eat, the feelings would still be there. So I let myself just feel those feelings, as hard as it was, and the next morning I had a better feeling."

One night, Jason and I were walking around in one of Chicago's well-known gay neighborhoods, and he was checking out other guys. He is a firm believer that when we are attracted to others and the eye wants to wander, it's natural to let it. Intellectually, I agree with him, but that night, it was difficult for me to watch, maybe because I was feeling insecure. I felt upset, but I just calmly said, "Hey, I am going home now." As I walked home, I thought I would go to Walgreens and buy circus peanuts or a bunch of Gummi bears, which I love. I was literally crying as I walked. I saw a pizza place and thought, "I'll just go eat a pizza." But I stopped myself. Deep down, I knew I wasn't really hungry. I felt hurt and scared and not good enough.

This time, instead of stuffing my face and my feelings, I tried to stay aware of those feelings. Then the lightbulb went on: whether I ate or didn't eat, the feelings would still be there. So I let myself just feel those feelings, as hard as it was, and the next morning I had a better feeling. It was Glory, Hallelujah! I got through that. No circus peanuts needed!

TAKE-AWAY: Feel the pain

If you're prone to eating when you're upset or angry, remember that food is not the answer. Instead of reaching for food, let yourself experience the emotions, knowing that they won't last forever.

Living through My Plateau

LaShon, 34, Virginia, emergency department nurse

In the beginning, it was easy. The weight just came off. I started Weight Watchers in January 2003, at 191 pounds. I am 5 feet 9 inches, and my goal was 147. By October, I was down to 159, and I was so happy. Just 12 pounds to go! The homestretch.

Then it hit. The plateau started before the holidays. October went by, November went by. I'd go up 2 pounds, down 2, but I had no real or lasting loss. I couldn't seem to make it out of the 150s. I was okay with it through the holidays. I figured, if I wasn't gaining, I should be happy. But then, after the first of the year, I got annoyed about the fact that I was just plain stuck.

And I was frustrated. So I took all the suggestions my leader and anyone else had for me about outwitting the plateau. I exercised more. I dropped down to a lower *POINTS* range for some days of the week.

But my weigh-ins remained the same. Up 2, down 2; the 150s seemed here to stay. For weeks it went like this. Weeks turned into months. For five long months, my weight did not budge except for those annoying 2-pound swings.

I decided to try to get through it. After all, I was close to my goal. I worked on being okay with this lack of progress by reminding myself, every time I was discouraged, that I had already made a lot of progress and I was not quitting now. I just kept thinking, "Well, 159 is a lot better than 191." I knew, deep down, that if I accepted the plateau, I would stick with it. I knew that if I didn't, I would quit in disgust. This probably sounds funny, but I started to embrace the plateau. To me, that didn't mean I loved the plateau, but I had to stop hating it.

When eating less and moving more didn't seem to work, I decided to work even more on my mental attitude, my plan to embrace this darn plateau. I also tried to keep things in perspective. My motto became "159 is better than 191." And that helped me to hang in there.

I had come way too far not to. I'd been a size 14 or 16 before, and the weight had just crept on. I used to eat all the wrong things, even though as a nurse I should have known better. After work, I'd often have fried chicken. I just didn't pay attention to my diet. For work, I wear scrubs, and they are so forgiving: you can put on 30 pounds and wear the same pair of scrubs. The tops are big, and they can hide a lot.

So I accepted the plateau, which meant I had to forget about feelings of disgust and frustration and focus on acceptance. I accepted where I was at the moment—and for the last five months—without questions or annoyance. I realized, "Isn't this part of life?" Whatever problem you have or bad habit you are dealing with, you have to step back and take stock, figure out where you are at the moment, how bad the problem is. Only then can you accept where you are and how much work you have to do. Only then can you move on to the next state—solving the problem or getting rid of the bad habit.

Just as I was getting really good at accepting the plateau, it disappeared. Just like that! By the end of February, I started to lose, little by little, until those last pounds were gone by March 2004. Actually, by March, I lost 14 more pounds, not just 12, getting down to 145, 2 pounds less than my goal. Since then, I have settled in at 147. That's a loss of 44 pounds. I like this weight.

I'm more careful now about what I eat. I had always exercised, but now I am more focused. I work three 12-hour shifts, so the days I have off, I work out. I run five miles, two or three times a week.

Now I wear a size 8, and my boyfriend Steve is always telling me I look hot. It's been more than three years since I reached my goal, and I still think about how glad I am to be off that plateau. But I am also grateful for my time spent on it because the plateau taught me so much—about patience, persistence, and just accepting yourself at a moment in time.

"When eating less and moving more didn't seem to work, I decided to work even more on my mental attitude. I also tried to keep things in perspective. My motto became '159 is better than 191.' And that helped me to hang in there."

TAKE-AWAY: Accept where you are now

When you feel discouraged by the rate—or lack—of progress you're experiencing, try to accept and appreciate yourself at your current weight. This can help you to hang in there until you begin losing again.

It's All about Portions

Susan, 43, New York, receptionist

The hardest part of losing weight was learning what a portion was. To me, when you got a package of cookies, the package was a portion. I remember as a kid, my mom and I would start at opposite ends of the ice cream box and meet in the middle. For most of my life, I was probably eating double to triple what I should have been eating at every meal. I mean, you would not be able to see the bottom of the plate when I put food on it.

I guess it's not surprising that I've pretty much been overweight all my life. But it got steadily worse when I got married and even worse after I had my son. Whatever he didn't eat, I ate because I didn't want it to go to waste.

Finally, I decided to do something about my weight. One morning at the end of December 2004, I was trying to put my pants on and they were just so tight. I was miserable. The night before, I'd got into bed and I wound up with these palpitations in my chest. I thought I was dying. I'm divorced, and my son is thirteen now. I knew I had to lose weight for myself but also to be around for him, to take care of him.

> "I remember as a kid, my mom and I would start at opposite ends of the ice cream box and meet in the middle."

In the past, I always used to say, "I'll start my diet on Monday." But Monday never comes. It just passes you by, then it's a month from now, and I'd say, "Okay, I'll start this Monday." And I never did.

That winter morning, I looked in the mirror and realized that I had to get a handle on my weight, that if I didn't do something about it, I was going to wind up dead. My blood pressure had already started to get out of control.

It took me just under two years to lose 77 pounds. In all that time, I never missed a Weight Watchers meeting. I also started to walk between two and four miles a day, do tai chi twice a week, and change what I ate. Now I eat more vegetables in a week than I have in the last thirty years. And now, when I serve myself food, you can actually see the plate underneath.

I've learned that you can eat everything—but just not in one day. The best weight-loss advice I ever heard was "One bite tastes like the rest." For my son's graduation, he wanted me to taste the cake so I took one forkful. He said, "That's all you're going to have?" and I said, "Now I know what it tastes like. I don't need any more." It has to be looked at one bite at a time, one portion at a time, one day at a time.

TAKE-AWAY: Savor the flavor

When you do indulge in a rich dessert or another high-calorie treat, eat it slowly and really enjoy the flavor; chances are, you'll feel satisfied after just a few bites and will be able to put down your fork or spoon.

Share, Share, Share

Think about which emotions trigger negative reactions that can and have sabotaged your weight-control efforts. Now think about alternative strategies for handling those emotions, then draw up a plan for what you'll do instead of using food as an emotional crutch in the future.

_____

_____

_____

_____

_____

_____

_____

_____

_____

_____

_____

_____

_____

CHAPTER 5

New Brides,
New Moms

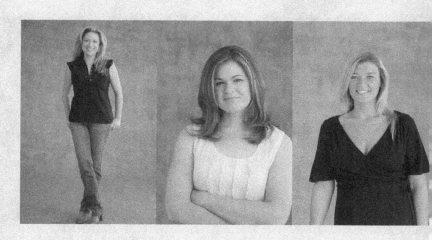

Whether you're facing the prospect of getting married or becoming a mother, you're sure to find yourself in the midst of an emotionally charged period of your life. In many ways, these can be the best of times and the worst of times as relationships and responsibilities shift. All of these issues can bring a woman's relationship with her body to center stage. The women featured in this chapter share their journeys through these life-altering transitions. You'll learn from their trials and tribulations—and discover new ways to navigate your own course through similar stages in your life.

The Incredible Shrinking Wedding Dress

Jessica, 30, New York, student and veterinary assistant

I had tried on about twenty-five wedding dresses and was getting discouraged. Nothing fit, nothing looked right. Then, at the third bridal shop, I finally found "The One."

It wasn't a traditional wedding dress. It was strapless and floor length, antique white with a burgundy leafy pattern across the bust. I loved it. And it would go perfectly with my fiancé Kamad's barong. It's a blousy, embroidered shirt, and it's traditional Filipino wedding attire for the groom.

My two aunts, who had come shopping with me, loved the dress, too. But there was a problem. The bridal shop only had it in a size 12, and it wouldn't zip up. The saleswomen had to hold it in the back for me so that I could see what it would look like if it fit.

I looked in the mirror and got tears in my eyes. Yes, the hunt was definitely over. I wanted to look beautiful at our wedding, to be the princess every woman wants to be. And this dress was definitely fit for a princess.

The saleswoman measured me, to see what size I needed. She said I needed a size 18, and I went ahead and ordered it. But I also told her I was going to lose a lot of weight before my wedding. This was January 2005, and the wedding was to be in October. She and the other salespeople just kind of nodded. I am sure they hear brides say that all the time. They said, "We'll have you in for another fitting and if we have to take it in, we will." I think they didn't really believe I would lose much.

I didn't tell them that I had joined Weight Watchers a few weeks earlier because a friend had lost weight on it. I had already lost about 8 pounds. Granted, I had a very long way to go. In January 2005, I had weighed in at 192—way too much for my height, 5 feet 1 inch. My doctor had suggested that 140 would be a good weight for me. So that was my goal, to lose 52 pounds.

About the same time, my three-year-old niece, Sunny, was visiting. Her mother had just had another baby, and Sunny looked at me, in the innocent way kids have, and said, "My mommy was real fat when my baby sister was in her belly." Then she said, "You look like you are fat enough to have a baby." Innocent as her comment was, it confirmed everything negative that I was feeling about myself at the time.

Losing weight wasn't just about the dress being a smaller size. I wanted to be able to enjoy my wedding day and be comfortable with my self-image. I didn't want to worry about looking fat. In the past, I worried about that all the time. My weight was such a huge burden emotionally; sometimes I would get in a horrible mood when I tried to find something to wear. Nothing looked good. So I committed myself to losing weight, and I lost a pound or 2 pounds every week.

The dress arrived in April. I had lost 37 pounds and was down to 155, just 15 pounds short of my goal. I was very excited as I went to the shop to try it on but was also nervous.

The saleswoman was amazed at how much weight I had lost. "This is way too big," she said. "You are swimming in it. We are going to have to send it back." She ordered a size 11, a junior size. It would take several months, again, to get the dress.

The second dress arrived in August. I got the call from the bridal shop right after I weighed in at 130, 10 pounds less than my goal. When I hit 140, I decided that I'd try to lose another 10, and it wasn't that difficult. I hurried down to the bridal shop to try it on. I went into the dressing room and slipped it on. My heart sank. The dress was beautiful but way too big, again. When I stepped out of the dressing room, the saleswomen had a look of horror on their faces. They knew there was not enough time to order a third dress. They were panicked. And so was I.

They took measurements and pinned the dress and called in their best seamstress. She had to alter this size-11 dress down to a size 6. She was afraid that it wouldn't look like the same dress, but she promised to do her best.

I was very nervous. I could have just found another dress that fit, but I wanted *that* dress and I wasn't giving up on that dress, just as I wasn't giving up on losing weight.

Two weeks before the wedding, the bridal shop called me for the final fitting. I was a nervous wreck. My maid of honor went with me. As I went into the dressing room, I had butterflies in my stomach. Then, once I got the dress on and zipped it up, I became completely calm. It fit perfectly. My maid of honor was beaming; she thought it looked perfect, too. The salespeople stepped in to admire it. One woman pulled aside other customers to tell them how much weight I had lost. At that point, I had lost 62 pounds.

Standing there, looking at myself in the mirror, I realized that this dress—and the weight loss that helped to make this dress look so beautiful—was everything I had wanted for so long. I was happy and really proud of myself.

I had not described the dress to Kamad because I wanted him to be surprised when he first saw me in it. He knew it needed to be altered, but that was it. He had helped me to lose weight by always offering to go jogging with me. We went bike riding together, too.

Our wedding was at Belhurst Castle in upstate New York, overlooking Seneca Lake. I had to walk down a long staircase to get to an archway with windows overlooking the lake. Kamad was standing under the archway. When he saw me, his eyes got bigger than I've ever seen. When I got closer, he leaned over and whispered in my ear, "You look beautiful." He said that many, many times that day.

"Losing weight wasn't just about the dress being a smaller size. I wanted to be able to enjoy my wedding day and be comfortable with my self-image, emotionally. I didn't want to worry about looking fat."

We have been married more than two years now. The wedding dress is tucked away in my closet. I get it out and look at it from time to time. I will probably try it on soon, but I know it will be too big because I've lost another 15 pounds. I weigh 115 now and wear a size 4. It's the thinnest I've been, by far, my entire adult life. Married life is wonderful. And these days, I never wake up in a horrible mood.

TAKE-AWAY: Boost your comfort quotient

Losing weight isn't only about enhancing how you look on the outside; it's also about improving how you feel in your own skin. Focusing on boosting that comfort quotient can keep you motivated throughout the weight-loss journey.

How I Stopped Hiding behind Eating

Monica, 26, New York, sixth-grade teacher

My lowest moment ever was trying on a wedding dress in a size 18 and seeing myself in the mirror. I thought, "Oh, no, I cannot get married like this." I was twenty-three and I weighed 200 pounds. I'm only 5 feet 2 inches.

When I was younger I was really just chubby. Then I went to college in New York City, where I studied acting, which is ironic because I'm very shy—and I gained weight. I had a couple of roommates who were skinny and gorgeous, and next to them I was the fat one. I felt out of place and I didn't have very many friends so I used food as a friend. Between classes I would go to the Mexican restaurant a block from the dorms and eat a huge plate of nachos. That would make me feel happy and comfortable for the moment, but, of course, I gained weight and then felt even more out of place.

I think I liked acting and singing because I could escape my shyness and transform myself into a happy, worry-free person. I didn't stand out as the pretty, confident girl that all of the boys liked, but I did stand out on stage. After auditions on campus, people who wouldn't normally talk to me would come over and tell me how great I'd been. It was a chance for me to shine when I had no other outlet to do so. When I wasn't acting, I felt invisible.

I had met my husband in college, and we later started living together in New York. I became a teacher at an elementary school, where I'm also the drama director. My husband never knew me thin so he didn't care about my weight. And I thought I didn't care much, either.

Looking back, it was as if I was walking around in a haze. I was always tired and often in pain, but I didn't realize that wasn't normal until after I'd lost the weight. I'd sometimes wonder what it would feel like to be the thin girl I always wanted to be, but I didn't think it could happen because I had too much weight to lose. I seemed happier to other people than I was—I was the jolly chubby person in public— but really I was painfully insecure. I was constantly embarrassed by my body. I felt like I took up too much space and that everybody was judging me, even if they weren't.

After my boyfriend and I got engaged and I tried on that size-18 wedding dress, I told my mother-in-law about wanting to lose weight, and she suggested that I come to a Weight Watchers meeting with her. I was so embarrassed about how I had looked in the dress that I was willing to do anything, but I wasn't optimistic. I just couldn't imagine eating healthy all the time or sitting in a room listening to other people talk about their weight. After the first time, it still felt a little weird, but I felt like, "Okay, maybe I can do this."

I now realize that healthy eating is a learned thing. So I made changes slowly, gradually cutting back on the amounts of sweets I ate or substituting things like yogurt, popcorn, and Jell-O for junky snacks. I did the same thing with fruit. At first I had to force myself, but gradually I came to really enjoy different fruits. Now they're a big part of my diet—strawberries and grapes are my favorites and I like that they're very filling.

Fast food was another story. I used to eat it every day. My husband and I would go into a fast-food place and split a twenty-piece box of chicken nuggets, then share an order of fajitas and fries. It was cheap, and because it tasted good, I felt happy while I was eating it. Unfortunately, it also made me want to eat more—as soon as I had something like that, I'd think about what else I could eat. So I knew I had to totally cut out fast food because I wouldn't be able to avoid overeating it. I haven't been into a fast-food place since I started to lose weight.

Aside from food itself, the biggest challenge was probably other people. When you're fat, people are constantly telling you to go on a diet. Then when you do start to lose weight, they try to get you to eat more, to cheat. They'll push food on you and say, "Oh come on, you can have a little." When I was invited to dinner, I used to dread having to tell people I was watching my weight and didn't want the cake, but I learned that the way not to hurt their feelings was to eat more of the healthy foods and tell them how good these were. If someone said, "You have to have some of this cake," I'd say, "You know, I'm really craving some of that delicious fruit salad you made. Can I have some?" Then I'd continue talking and lead the conversation in a different direction.

By our wedding date, November 12, 2005, I had lost 70 pounds. It was so exciting. When I went back for a fitting, I had to reorder the dress in a size 8; the girls in the shop could barely believe I had lost so much weight. The wedding was fun. There were many people who had not seen me since I'd lost the weight, and they were shocked. It felt great to see their reactions. It was what I had been dreaming about for so many years. So was our honeymoon in Aruba. We did all kinds of things I would never have thought I could do before, like wearing a swimsuit, jet-skiing, and riding an ATV.

After the wedding I had about 10 more pounds to lose, and it was different because before, imagining myself as a thin bride had been my motivation. As I continued to lose, and now that I'm on maintenance, it's enough to remember how I was before—how I felt invisible, as if people wouldn't notice me when I walked into a store or waited in line. Being heavy was like being stuck in the shadows, and losing the weight helped me to step into the spotlight and stop hiding behind eating and my fat. I never want to be that way again.

> "I made changes slowly, gradually cutting back on the amounts of sweets I ate or substituting things like yogurt, popcorn, and Jell-O for junky snacks. I did the same thing with fruit. At first I had to force myself, but gradually I came to really enjoy different fruits."

Now that I've lost 80 pounds—I weigh 120—I no longer feel invisible or self-conscious. I feel energized and like the world is open to me in a way it wasn't before. Losing weight has given me a sense of freedom and adventure that I hope to have for the rest of my life.

TAKE-AWAY: Stand up to food pushers

Whenever a host pressures you to eat something you'd like to avoid at a social gathering, tell her you'll either try it later or that what you really have your eye on is another (healthier) dish on the table. Complimenting a food pusher on something she's offering will distract her from her agenda and help you to stick with yours.

Cooking and Eating Great Food—the Healthy Way

Nicola, 32, New York, fashion and event publicist

I have my own company in New York City doing publicity for small fashion designers and events like movie premieres. I'm constantly surrounded by beautiful people and clothes, so in 2006, when I found myself with 30 extra pounds that I just couldn't get rid of after I had my baby, I felt like the ugly duckling. Up until then, I'd always had what I consider a good body. I was never skinny—I always had the boobs and the butt, but I was fine with that, and I was always self-confident. I was raised that way.

I grew up in Ireland with three sisters and two brothers, and my mother taught us to have a healthy relationship with food and our bodies. My mother was skinny 'til her fifth baby, and then she started putting on a little weight, but she still always looked amazing. She always had her hair done and her lipstick on, and she never went out in slippers like the other moms.

It was the same story with food. My mother was a phenomenal cook and threw weekly dinner parties. We used to regularly come home to the smell of homemade bread and soup cooking. There were never any negatives associated with food—it was just something to be enjoyed, and I did enjoy it! As a result, I don't get any pleasure out of grabbing a slice of pizza or fast food for dinner—I like meals to be something special. Of course, when I moved here in 1994, when I was eighteen, I was an au pair, so for the first few years all that I cooked and ate was kid food. But then I met my husband after just two months, and much of our courtship revolved around eating out. We loved splurging on gorgeous restaurants and discovered New York together through the entire dining experience.

After we'd been together for about five years, we began to settle down and cook at home, instead. For the first time, I really looked at the foods in the grocery store and was amazed by the freshness. In Ireland, vegetables come wrapped in cellophane, and it's hard to get really fresh fish anymore, even though it's an island. Most of Ireland's fish is exported. Here, every corner grocery store has fresh veggies on ice, and I can stop at the fish market on my way home from work. Everything is so beautifully presented that I just want to buy and cook it!

I had my first daughter in 2003, and after she was born, the weight came off pretty easily. But after my second pregnancy, three years later, I was stuck with about 30 pounds that just wouldn't come off. Gaining that weight was the only thing that had ever attacked my self-confidence. It's important to me not to have any negative issues around food and body image in my house, especially now that I have children. In my four-year-old daughter's class recently I heard one of the little girls say, "I'm fat," and you know she picked that up at home. So when I started to feel myself getting negative, I knew it was a problem.

> "Instead of heavy cream sauces—I was experimenting with Italian food after the baby was born and was doing big pots of cheesy pasta for dinner—I'll sauté some shrimp in a fresh basil and tomato sauce and serve it with whole-wheat pasta."

I don't want to be skinny; I just want to be strong and fit. I want to be able to wear a gorgeous dress on the red carpet. I want to be able to pick up my four-year-old if she needs that. When I walk outside, I don't want to be picking and pulling at my clothes, but I've found that when you're heavy, nothing fits right, even in a bigger size.

My sisters in Ireland had done Weight Watchers to lose their post-pregnancy weight, so when I realized I was really struggling with mine, I joined here in Brooklyn. I went to the meetings religiously, I became more aware of high-calorie foods, and I gained the willpower to say no to something when it wasn't what I really craved anyway. I physically can't force myself to buy a bag of chips anymore, knowing how many calories are in it!

It was a relief to figure out that I didn't have to give up cooking and eating great food to lose the weight—I just had to tone down the rich ingredients a little. For example, we used to have cheese and crackers before dinner—now we might have oysters. Instead of heavy cream sauces—I was experimenting with Italian food after the baby was born and was doing big pots of cheesy pasta for dinner—I'll sauté some shrimp in a fresh basil and tomato sauce and serve it with whole-wheat pasta. I still use the time spent cooking dinner as my way to relax after a long day at work. I might pick up fish and veggies on the way home and grill the kids a simple dinner. After they're in bed, my husband and I will pour a glass of wine and have a great meal together. Right now I'm into big, spicy stir-fries with tons of vegetables, served over a small portion of egg noodles. I like to make us several light courses instead of one big one and to present the food in the middle of a big, white, restaurant-style plate—I find that eating with your eyes makes you actually consume less!

It feels so good to be thin again. I firmly believe that when you have self-confidence, you radiate that. People flock to you, and good things come to you. I have way too busy and happy a life to spend time moping over how I look. Now I can just pop out of the house without worrying about my body the way I used to. And I don't spend all spring dreading the weddings that I'll have to dress up for and the beach outings I need to buy a bathing suit for. Life is easier now! For my family and myself, every day is an adventure, and I'm not going to waste it worrying about my looks.

TAKE-AWAY: Focus on the presentation

If you arrange your food creatively on the center of a plate with a large rim, you'll be giving your eyes and mind a real treat—and you'll be practicing portion control at the same time.

Getting My Body Ready
for Baby

. . . .

Tina, 40, Georgia, real estate attorney

In September 2005, when I was thirty-eight, my husband and I decided to visit an ob-gyn to talk about family planning. We weren't ready to start having kids yet, but we wanted to set the groundwork and see whether there was anything we should be doing to get our bodies ready. I figured she'd tell me to drink more milk or juice. So when she said, "You need to lose weight. In your current state of obesity you would pose a health problem to your unborn child," I thought, "Oh, my God!"

I'd been heavy for awhile, but I had never thought of myself as obese. Obese people had to stay at home, they couldn't lead normal lives, their daily actions were restricted, whereas I was completely healthy—or so I believed. Every year I religiously had my annual check-up, and every year I got what I considered a clean bill of health. The doctor would say, "You don't have the Big Three: diabetes, high cholesterol, or high blood pressure. You're relatively healthy. But . . . you should lose weight." I never heard anything after the word *healthy*.

I never felt ashamed or guilty for being overweight, which is part of the reason I was able to ignore my weight for so long. My husband didn't worry about my weight either because all he cared about was that I was happy. But after that ob-gyn appointment, for the first time he sat down with me and said, "Maybe we should do something about your weight." At first I resisted, but within the same month, another thing happened to make me face the reality that my obesity was affecting my life. I was wriggling into my control-top pantyhose one morning before work when I had to stop and sit down and rest with my stockings around my knees. My heart was racing. I had broken into a sweat. I was exhausted. "What's happening to me?" I thought. It took me three tries to get those pantyhose up. That was my lightbulb moment.

I started to see the truth. I used to think my weight didn't affect me, but once I thought about it, I realized there were lots of times when I decided not to go out with my girlfriends after work because I was too tired. I didn't have the energy to go clothes shopping at the mall anymore, and even if I did, I couldn't wear any of the cute clothes. I didn't have the energy to pick up groceries after work. An eight-hour workday was as much as I could handle. And now I couldn't even get myself dressed in the morning. How did I think I was going to get up for midnight feedings or chase a toddler around? Suddenly, it all became perfectly clear. I told my husband, "You're right, my weight is a problem."

I suggested surgery because I'd been on too many diets in my life, and I'd tried to exercise and always failed after three days. But my husband wanted me to try Weight Watchers. I wasn't shy or anything; I just didn't like the idea of people telling me what to eat. But I made a deal with my husband. I'd try Weight Watchers, and if it didn't work, we'd consider surgery. If I lost even 1 pound the first week, I'd continue.

So I went to my first At Work meeting, and the first thing I heard was, "You can eat anything you want." That got my attention. I really worked hard that first week because I wanted to be able to say to my husband with all honesty that I tried my hardest and it didn't work. And when I stepped on the scale and saw that I had lost weight, I was shocked and amazed. It challenged everything I thought I knew about "dieting" because I felt that I had eaten whatever I wanted—though not in the same quantities—and I lost weight! I reported back to my husband, and he was like, "Okay, we're in."

"Every single day for sixteen months, while I was losing, I had a slice of Weight Watchers Double Fudge Chocolate Cake at night, and looking forward to that gave me the strength to resist the Krispy Kremes or pizza at work."

He remained my partner in this every step of the way—every food choice, every portion, every page of my food journal. He would come grocery shopping with me and say, "Do you want these vegetables?

What about these?" When I told him we couldn't buy all these fruits and vegetables because there wasn't enough room in the fridge, he had a wall knocked out and installed a commercial fridge for me!

Every now and then I'd get to feeling self-pity. I'd think, "Why do I have to stop at one piece of pizza instead of being able to eat the whole thing like other people?" Then I'd remind myself that no one was forcing this on me; it was my journey, my choices, my reality. To keep from feeling deprived, I also made sure that I always had one really good "daily indulgence." Every single day for sixteen months, while I was losing, I had a slice of Weight Watchers Double Fudge Chocolate Cake at night, and looking forward to that gave me the strength to resist the Krispy Kremes or pizza at work.

One thing I did not do, and this sets me apart from many people, is exercise. I had so many bad associations with exercise. I used to hold myself up to high standards, and if I couldn't do half an hour on the treadmill, as I had done when I was eighteen, I'd consider myself a failure. Every year, I'd rejoin the gym and buy new workout clothes, and I always gave up after three days. After I started losing weight, it took a while for me to readjust my idea of what movement could be, to accept that this is my journey to make in my own way and I didn't have to stand up to anyone else's standards. I still can't do even fifteen minutes on the treadmill, but I hike and do belly dancing, and I carry forty-pound bags of topsoil around my yard. I'm proud of that.

I lost 95 pounds and reached my goal in March 2007. Now, having a family is an option for us. I feel such a sense of relief in other ways, too. I feel like I can finally be myself—I can go out to dinner with my friends after work or shop in any store in the mall, not just in the plus-size shop way in the back. But the real thing I've accomplished is achieving a healthy lifestyle. I remember the day I lost my last pound, I said to myself, "I am no longer a health statistic!" For the first time in my life, when people talk about the obesity epidemic in America, I am not a part of it. That makes me feel wonderful.

TAKE-AWAY: Cancel the pity party

When you start to feel sorry for yourself about your weight, remind yourself that most people face personal struggles during their lifetimes—and it's your choice whether to do something about yours.

Bouncing Back after Baby

Jenny McCarthy, 36, California, actor, author

I gained nearly 90 pounds during my pregnancy. I was eating everything! For breakfast I'd have eggs Benedict with hash browns and bacon; a couple of hours later I'd have a tuna sandwich with onion rings; an hour after that I'd gulp down a milkshake and a hot dog. For dinner I'd have a slab of ribs, a baked potato, and beans. I'd finish it off with a pan of brownies! Eventually, I stopped weighing myself and wouldn't let my doctor tell me my weight!

When I checked in at the hospital to have my son, a nurse practically screamed my weight over the loudspeaker. She said to an assistant, "She's 211!" I was like, "Nooooo!" I was horrified! Later, two of my sisters walked into my house and found me sitting there in a near stupor, wearing only my giant bra and underpants. I was just crying, "Ohmigod, ohmigod!" To get motivated, I went into my bathroom, took off all my clothes, stood on top of the toilet, and looked at my fat in the mirror under the fluorescent lights. I stared at it. I shook it. I squeezed it. Finally, I said to myself, "Oh, this is bad!" Each butt cheek was four times its pre-baby size! The cellulite hung down my thighs and over my kneecaps. My waist had a tire around it.

"My sister was my most enthusiastic cheerleader. We joined together so we encouraged each other along the way. I recommend joining with someone!"

First I tried the Hollywood thing: I hired the best personal trainer, and I did one hour of cardio every day, plus three days a week of weight training. After one month, I hadn't lost a pound! And I was starving myself, eating only peas and sashimi! That just goes to show you need to eat consistently to keep your metabolism moving. After a month of torture, I called my mom, crying. Mom said she'd just lost a lot of weight on Weight Watchers. I thought, "I'm the one in Hollywood. How can I take my mother's advice on dieting?" But I didn't know what else to do so I found a meeting. And as long as there were no photographers, I felt comfortable with others who were struggling with their weight. Other members recognized me, but that didn't matter. A camaraderie developed, and we cheered one another on.

During my first six months on the program, I lost a good deal of weight. I started out as a size 12 or 14; I got down to a 6, and now I'm back in a 4.

My sister was my most enthusiastic cheerleader. We joined together so we encouraged each other along the way. I recommend joining with someone! It helped me so much.

TAKE-AWAY: Practice mindful eating

Turn off the automatic pilot and make it a policy to always be truly conscious of what and how much you're putting in your mouth.

Visualize the Future

If you frequently imagine how being thin will enhance the experiences you want to have with your friends, your loved ones, or on your own, you'll probably find it easier to beat temptation when it strikes. What other ways can you think of to be kind to yourself?

_____

_____

_____

_____

_____

_____

_____

_____

_____

_____

_____

_____

CHAPTER 6

Embracing Challenge

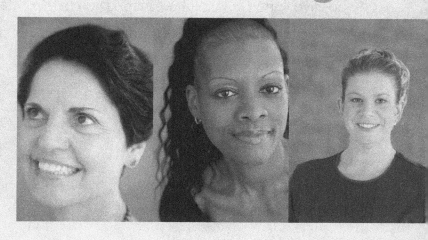

Have you ever watched runners crossing the finish line at a marathon and thought, "Wow—I could never do that!"? In this chapter, you'll read about people who were in a similar place but proved themselves wrong. As they pushed themselves to get out of their comfort zones, many of them discovered passions for new forms of movement or found a level of mental and physical fortitude they didn't know they had. Along the way, they came to see themselves in a stronger, more positive light. Their spirit will inspire you to think clearer, act smarter, and take worthy chances as you set off on the path to becoming the healthier person you really want to be.

Losing Weight, Finding My Sisters

Dawn, 38, Maryland, marketing coordinator for a real estate firm

The idea hit me one day in September 2005 when I was having my nails done. I saw a flyer for something called Team in Training. It said they would train you, for free, to do a marathon in Arizona to raise money for charity. I admit that at first my motives were all selfish. I thought, "Hey, I'll get a mini-vacation to Phoenix and a free trainer, and I can finally lose some weight!" Then when I saw that it was to raise money for leukemia, I knew that I had to do it. That's what my sister Diane died of fifteen years ago when she was only twenty-seven.

First, I called the organizers, whom I knew because my dad organizes golf tournaments for leukemia research. I said, "You know how heavy I am. Be honest—can I do this?" When they said yes, I pretty much went down there and signed up on the spot. I'd always been chunky, and I'd tried a thousand diets. But when I signed up for this race, I knew that there was no way I was going to be able to do it without losing some weight. So I knew I'd have to improve my eating habits, too.

When I told my mom I was going to do the marathon, she told my older sister Debbie, who called me and basically said, "I want to do it, too!" So I sent her the information, and two weeks later we showed up together on a Saturday morning for our first training session.

After Diane died, Debbie and I kind of grew apart. We lived in the same town, but we probably only saw each other every six weeks or so. We just had very different lives—I'm married and have two kids; she and her husband are very close, have no kids, and are really into horseback riding. We just figured we had nothing in common so a distance grew between us.

But we discovered that we did have something in common: we both wanted to do something to keep Diane's memory alive. What happened between Debbie and me during this process was wonderful—we realized that not only do we love each other because we're sisters, but we really like each other! I got to know who she really is, and we became best friends. For that reason alone, it was worth it.

As a side benefit, we got in shape together. Without Debbie cheering me on, I could never have done the training. We'd meet three days a week at 6 a.m. to walk at a track near our homes, and on Saturdays we'd train with the Leukemia and Lymphoma Society people.

In the beginning I could barely walk twenty minutes because I was so overweight. I'm really laid back and probably would have just given up, but Debbie does things 100 percent. She's a total optimist and she kept me going. When I was tired, she'd say, "Think about Diane. Think about how much pain she must have been in at the hospital. You can walk one hour for her, two hours, three hours!" I'd be looking at her with dagger eyes, but she'd be right there behind me, urging me on.

It was an emotional journey because it was a total dedication to Diane's memory. There were many Saturdays when, if I hadn't had the memory of her to keep me going, I would have stopped. Diane was the rocket in our family, so full of life and pizzazz—it would have been fun to do this race with her. We would have laughed our way through the whole thing! There isn't a day that I don't think of her or of something I'd like to say to her. She's really my inspiration.

> "What happened between Debbie and me during this process was wonderful—we realized that not only do we love each other because we're sisters, but we really like each other! I got to know who she really is, and we became best friends."

Thanks to her, I've turned my life around and made it healthier. I know that I will continue to walk and run marathons for the rest of my life because it's part of who I am now. It feels incredible to be fit and thin! I'm also more positive in general. These days, it takes a lot for me to get upset because I'm clear about what matters most—for me, it's family.

I'd like to think that we took something tragic and turned it into something good. I have only one sister left, and I want to make the best of that relationship.

TAKE-AWAY: Treat yourself like an athlete

Start exercising regularly and taking care of yourself as if you are an athlete—by fueling yourself with healthy, energy-boosting foods and plenty of sleep—and you'll likely lose weight more easily.

Sticking with It

Catherine, 50, Louisiana, senior administrative assistant

The hardest part of my weight-loss journey was being evacuated by Hurricane Katrina with only 10 pounds to go until I reached my goal weight. I was forty-five when I decided to lose weight. I had always been heavy—my daughter and my grandson had never known me any other way. I got heavy in high school. I had a hearing problem and I was shy, so I just stayed home and ate. Then I had my daughter, and life as a single mother was really tough. I was so busy, plus I was working at Burger King, so that's all I ate. I kept gaining weight, but, to be honest, I didn't care. My priority was just raising my daughter.

When she was three or four, I got a job at the place I work now, the local utility company—I've been here for twenty-four years. My boss and dear friend Tina was a Weight Watchers member, and in April 2003 she asked me to come with her. I didn't want to—I thought I had too much weight to lose—but she said, "This isn't about your weight; it's about your health." I was almost 300 pounds by this time, and I thought about how much my knees and back hurt, how I got out of breath walking short distances, and how it broke my heart when my two-year-old grandson asked me to get down on the floor and play with him and I couldn't. So I went.

It was hard the first day. But I just looked around, saw that everyone else was in the same boat as me, and never turned back. And little by little, I realized it wasn't as hard as I thought. The hardest habits to break were the fried seafood—we just love that here in Louisiana—and soda. But as soon as I cut out the fried stuff and started to drink more water, I felt so much healthier, and that kept me going.

I thought it would take five years to lose 100 pounds, but in one year and eight months, by August 2005, I had lost 140! No one could believe it—not me, not my daughter. And then on August 29, when I had 10 pounds to go until my goal, the hurricane hit.

My house was in a town called Slidell, half an hour outside New Orleans, on Lake Pontchartrain. I lived there with my seventy-four-year-old mother, my daughter, and my grandson. Everyone knew the hurricane was coming our way, so we were evacuated to Montgomery, Alabama, 285 miles away. It was so nerve-wracking. For four or five days we had no phone contact with most of my family, including some of my brothers and sisters and my daughter, who was away in Baton Rouge; her son was with me.

After eleven days we were allowed to go back to our house in Slidell, although the power didn't come back on for a few days longer. We were really lucky—we didn't have much damage. But the building I worked in, in New Orleans, was flooded out, so my company relocated me and a good five hundred other employees to Jackson, Mississippi. They found us apartments and paid for the move. All we had to pay for was food. But it was sad because it wasn't home, and I had to leave my mother, my daughter, and my grandson back in Slidell. What made it a little easier was knowing they weren't all alone. My brother, his wife, and their four children, who lost everything in the hurricane, moved into our house until they bought their own place down the block the following year.

After about two months, I decided that I needed to get back on track with my weight loss. People might think weight is insignificant compared to a hurricane, but I had changed my life. I was a happier, healthier person after losing weight, and I was not going to ruin what I had started. No storm in the world could have made me do that. So I went to a meeting in Jackson, but it just didn't click. I needed to be with people who had gone through what I had in the hurricane. So I got off at two on Fridays and drove three hours each way to an evening meeting in Metairie, right near New Orleans, every week for the next six months. I belong with these people. Some of them have lost everything, and they're still here, working at getting healthy. We're like a family.

Once I started up at Weight Watchers again, it was so different from the way it was before the hurricane. Before, I attended an At Work meeting, and everything was so convenient and comfortable—I knew the people, I had the routine of work-meeting-home. Now, nothing was convenient. I felt as if my whole world had collapsed. My easy daily routine was gone, I had no family around me for support, I had to drive hours to my meeting, and I had to witness the pure devastation around me every Friday when I went back to New Orleans. But it was really important to me to finish, so I decided to make the best of the situation. I got used to the long drive and ended up using it to catch up with family, and even to talk on my cell phone with my leader, Theresa, whom I'd become good friends with.

Finally, in May 2006, nine months after I was relocated, our company moved back to New Orleans, and I moved back to my house in Slidell. But even though I no longer had to drive that long distance every week, emotionally, it was even harder after I got home. The aftermath of the hurricane is still going on down here, and the stress level is very high. Coming back after nine months, I hadn't had time to heal as other people had, so it was still fresh for me. Every day I drove through New Orleans and relived the hurricane and the evacuation all over again. I saw the neighborhood I grew up in, and nothing was there anymore. The crime was higher. The stores had long lines, and many businesses were closed. Work was also tough because we were all readjusting to being back together again. Another hard thing was coming from living alone to a house full of people—ten in all. I had all these other people's needs to think about, too, and the house was full of junk food.

"The hardest habits to break were the fried seafood—we just love that here in Louisiana—and soda. But as soon as I cut out the fried stuff and started to drink more water, I felt so much healthier, and that kept me going."

All of these things made me feel overwhelmed or down sometimes, and my first instinct was often to reach for something salty and eat a whole bag of chips. What I do now is stop and remember to focus on me and on the positive changes I have made. Sometimes I'll call a friend and talk it through. I also keep going to my meetings. Some of the other members think of me as an inspiration, so if I drop out, I feel like I'm letting them down, too. I reached my goal weight three days before Christmas 2006.

I am very proud of myself for continuing what I started when it would have been so easy to give up. I always remind myself that yes, a hurricane hit my town and devastated my life, but that is no excuse to let weight or bad health get the best of me. I'm worth more than that.

TAKE-AWAY: Hang out with people who inspire you

Whether you get practical tips from them or their can-do spirit simply bolsters your resolve, their healthy habits are bound to rub off on you in ways that will help you to pursue your goals.

Becoming a Cowgirl

Stacey, 41, Kansas, home-schooling mom to four kids

My husband jokes that I'm his cowgirl. I love horseback riding, and I've even ridden in four rodeos with my daughter—something I never would have done a few years ago. My horse's name is Dallas; he's nineteen years old, short and stocky and not terribly speedy, but he's a really wonderful boy and will do just about anything I ask him to. When I ride in a rodeo, I'm definitely nervous, but I feel strong, confident, and excited, too. The horse is running about forty miles per hour, and I don't have a lot of time to think. I do barrel racing, which is basically riding around barrels in a cloverleaf pattern, making loops. It's a blast! There is a certain adrenaline rush. I can't imagine myself ever skydiving or bungee jumping, but riding horses gives me a thrill.

When I was heavy, I wouldn't have even tried horseback riding because I would have thought, "Oh, the poor horse, with all that weight on it!" For years, my weight went up and down a lot, and it seemed like I was always trying to lose 5, 10, or 15 pounds. But I was never really, really heavy until after my second child. My weight got really low after my fourth child, then I gained it all back—with interest!—and maxed out at about 185. I'm 5 feet 2 inches.

I decided to do something about it because my cholesterol was high, my blood pressure was high, and I was probably headed for diabetes because I had gestational diabetes with my second pregnancy. And I just couldn't keep up with my four kids. I'd get out of breath doing little things like climbing stairs, folding laundry, even saying our nightly prayers with the kids! I just didn't like the way I looked or felt.

I used to do triathlons, and I taught aerobics classes. But after having kids, I had turned into a slug because I thought I was too busy to exercise. And I've always liked food a lot—pizza, popcorn, cookies—and I could put away a lot in one sitting. I just like the tastes, the way food feels in my mouth. And I love to bake. Homemade bread—oh, my goodness! I could eat a whole loaf of bread straight out of the oven.

After I found Weight Watchers Online, I started in February 2005. My husband is in the army, and he's gone a lot. I do a lot of volunteering for other army families whose husbands work for my husband, and I home-school our kids, who are now sixteen, fourteen, nine, and eight. The online plan was great for me. It really helped to write things down and see exactly what was going into my mouth.

One of the biggest changes is that I started to eat fruits and vegetables. I used to go for days without a fruit or a vegetable passing my lips. I didn't hate them, but I usually didn't feel like eating them. Another change was cheese—I used to eat a ton of it. I decided that I'd better not eat quite that much. Nowadays, I eat oatmeal for breakfast pretty much every day. I don't eat as much meat as I used to, and now I eat leaner meat—a lot of chicken, turkey, fish, pork tenderloins. At dinner, about half of my plate is now veggies, with a smaller portion of meat and a smaller portion of pasta.

In the past, my weak point was all-or-nothing thinking: either I was totally in control and eating very restrictively or else I was completely out of control and eating everything. There was no happy medium. Everything was a good food or a bad food. I hadn't figured out a way to eat that was livable. I probably was pretty close to my goal weight before I realized that I could do this and it didn't have to be this crazy, restrictive plan. That's when I knew this was something I could live with. These days, I still eat treats. I have pizza or cookies or ice cream sometimes, although I do eat less and plan for it. I'm a firm believer in eating everything—just not all at once and not in massive quantities.

> "I don't eat as much meat as I used to, and now I eat leaner meat—a lot of chicken, turkey, fish, pork tenderloins. At dinner, about half of my plate is now veggies, with a smaller portion of meat and a smaller portion of pasta."

As I was losing weight, I got back into exercising. I had already been walking; then I ramped it up to running. Next, I tried horseback riding and started to ride in rodeos.

Doing Weight Watchers, I lost 50 pounds and I reached 120 in September 2005. My husband was in Iraq while I lost most of the weight. He told me it was a good thing I had the kids with me at the airport because otherwise he wouldn't have recognized that it was me. He just kept turning and staring at me.

After losing weight, I just feel so much better about myself. I feel more confident. I can move around better. It's not just physically feeling better. I'm happier, too. I remember catching a glimpse of myself in a mirror in a store and thinking, "Wow! I'm beautiful." I'd never thought that before in my life. Cute? Sure, but never beautiful. It just feels so good now, and I love being attractive for my husband. He loves me anyway, but I know he certainly prefers me to look like this. He says I'm hotter now than I was at eighteen. I'll take it.

TAKE-AWAY: Fill half your plate with vegetables

The high water and fiber content of veggies can help to fill you up for relatively few calories and *POINTS* values, leaving room for high-quality protein, fruits, or grains on the other half of your plate.

Getting Back
into Exercise

Nazalee, 37, Ohio, fund-raiser for a major medical center

No one would have believed it, but back when I was a marathon runner, although I was thin, I was actually far less healthy than I am now. I had been an athlete all my life, running cross-country in high school and college. When I was in my twenties and living in Washington, D.C., I started to run marathons as a way to challenge myself. I was only into running, nothing else. In fact, I was a stuck-up runner. If I saw someone walking, I'd look down on her, thinking, "Oh, she's not really getting a workout."

Then, in 1999, I had to have minor surgery on my tailbone, probably as a result of too much running, and the doctor's orders were no running for three months. I was very upset. I could have walked or done yoga or Pilates, but for me, it was running or nothing. So that's what I did—nothing. I was stuck in a black-or-white state of mind, with no gray area in between, which is why I ended up gaining weight.

After the three-month period was up, I had gained about 20 pounds and didn't think I could run like I used to. I guess I also felt burned out, which I now know is the danger of the all-or-nothing attitude. So I continued to be a couch potato.

Unfortunately, I didn't change my eating habits. Even during my marathon days, I had never known how to eat right, although back then I could eat anything and not gain weight. I used to get all my meals out. I would have a sausage and egg muffin for breakfast, then a pre-made salad with tons of mayonnaise in the dressing for lunch. After 5 p.m. I'd stop by a bakery and buy four of the 50 percent–off cookies and eat them all. Dinner might be take-out fast food, lobster bisque, or fish and chips. I continued to eat like this after my surgery, so no wonder I started to gain weight.

As I gained, I knew I wasn't living healthily, but my tunnel vision kept me from doing anything about it. Because I felt fat, I looked at food as something bad, something I needed to try to burn off or feel guilty about. If I ate too much for lunch, I'd just call it a throwaway day and keep eating. If I had one cookie, I may as well have four—that kind of thing. I gained about 40 pounds a year for three years in a row—and got up to 272.

The final blow was when I had to get the same pants altered several times because I kept ripping the waistband—and it was elastic, not even zip-up. So I decided it was time to take charge. When I joined Weight Watchers in 2002, the hardest part was not looking at my weight-loss goal in one big lump, which was way too overwhelming. Instead, I made 10 percent increment goals. I didn't lose anything my first week on the program, which is unusual. I wanted to quit, but my leader took my hands and said, "You can do it. I want to see you back here next week." When I lost my first 5 pounds after a month, I cried. I had learned that there is a gray area in between fat and thin. Five pounds was a very good beginning.

I slowly started to get back into exercise. It was hard in the beginning, with my all-or-nothing mind-set, and as someone who had run marathons, I was embarrassed to be so out of shape. I wanted to say, "If I can't run six miles, then forget it, I'd rather do nothing." But I forced myself to accept that walking just twenty minutes was an acceptable compromise. Twenty minutes slowly became half an hour, and that became forty-five minutes, and so on. Whenever my current workout became too easy, I'd make it a little bit longer or harder.

> "Just as with exercise, eating any food to the extreme is bad—everything should be in moderation. Now I eat chocolate every day, but I make sure it's good, dark chocolate, and because I don't feel guilty, I'm able to stop after one piece."

After losing 30 pounds, I joined a gym, which was a mortifying experience at first. I felt that everyone was looking at me and thinking I didn't belong. But I focused on the happy feeling that exercise gave me and the way I worked out all the day's problems and left them on the machine.

Now I think of exercise as if it's a relationship—you have to keep it alive, varied and vibrant, or it will stagnate. I cross-train, which keeps me from getting bored and tones different muscles. I love Spinning, and I also do yoga and Pilates and take dancing lessons—tango is my favorite.

Before, I wouldn't let myself miss a complete workout because I thought if I slipped just a little, I'd quit altogether. Now I give myself the ten-minute rule: if I go to the gym and after ten minutes I still don't feel like being there, I leave. I almost never leave, but I always reserve the right!

As I got more in tune with my body, I learned to embrace the gray area in terms of eating, too. The dieting mentality—no dessert allowed; if you "cheat," then you've shot your day—is a recipe for crashing and burning. I lost almost 130 pounds, and I've kept it off for three years by looking at food not as good versus bad, allowed versus forbidden, but as something I need to nourish myself. Just as with exercise, eating any food to the extreme is bad—everything should be in moderation. Now I eat chocolate every day, but I make sure it's good, dark chocolate, and because I don't feel guilty, I'm able to stop after one piece. Now that food isn't the enemy anymore, eating is one of my favorite activities. I like to go to organic markets and discover new foods and put meals together myself.

By trying new things and learning that I can bend the rules, I've made my life less rigid and a lot happier. I've discovered that the gray zone is actually a rainbow of many different shades.

TAKE-AWAY: Try the ten-minute rule

Even if you really don't feel like exercising on a particular day, hit the trail, the court, or the gym for just ten minutes and give yourself permission to quit if you really want to after that. Chances are, you won't.

Riding for My Life

Peggy, 57, Ohio, special accounts manager for an insurance company

I'll never forget the moment I realized I was fat. It was July 2004, and I was at the Cedar Point Amusement Park in Sandusky, Ohio, not far from where I keep a boat. I had stopped by to ride the Millennium, the park's new roller coaster, on my way home from boating, and the young man who was operating the ride said I might not be able to go because the seat belt didn't have enough slack in it. He actually got out a tape measure and measured the seat belt. It was awful. Up until then, I'd thought of myself as someone who was a little heavy. I weighed 180 pounds.

My weight sort of crept up on me over the years. I gained a couple of pounds a year starting in my mid-thirties. I'd honestly never thought much about it because it had never stopped me from doing anything I wanted to do. I golfed and wore attractive clothes and enjoyed my life. But in that humiliating moment on that roller coaster it dawned on me: I'd become a fat old lady.

Not long after that, a friend at work said she was thinking about joining Weight Watchers, and I told her I'd go with her. She kept hemming and hawing, though, so I finally went without her. Everything I heard in that meeting kind of stuck with me. We were talking about how hard it is to socialize when you're watching what you eat, and the meeting leader said you just have to remind yourself that it's not about the food. That became a mantra of mine. I'd go out after work with friends for beer and tacos, but I'd tell myself it's not about the food, it's about hanging out with my friends. I do a lot of socializing, and a lot of my weight gain was from social drinking and eating out, so that mantra works for me to this day.

By February 2005 I reached my goal of 150 pounds, but I was worried about maintaining it. The biggest struggle for me is keeping my focus. It's so easy to stop thinking about what I'm eating or drinking. But every time I do that, the pounds creep back on.

Then in the spring of that year I had a life-changing event. My father's wife gave me her old road bike. I'd never ridden a bike more than a mile or two, but I thought it sounded like fun. I live close to a bike trail that runs along the Rocky River, and it's beautiful. So I started to go out every day, and I'd just ride farther and farther.

A couple of months later a friend asked me to participate in a thirty-mile ride on the Fourth of July. After I accepted, I thought, "What am I, crazy?" I'd never ridden more than five miles! I had no comprehension of what it would be like to ride thirty. But I felt sort of obligated to go since I said I would, so I went on the ride. There was a huge group of people, as it turned out, and everyone was just as nice as they could be. It was such a wonderful community, and that completely hooked me.

> "We were talking about how hard it is to socialize when you're watching what you eat, and the meeting leader said you just have to remind yourself that it's not about the food. That became a mantra of mine."

The ride was surprisingly easy for me, and when we got home I was so darn proud of myself. I was fifty-three years old and thought, "Wow, how could I wait so long to do something like that?" Anyway, the ride was put on by a biking group called the Lake Erie Wheelers, and I decided to join up. I began to ride with them regularly, and I rode on my own every day that I wasn't with them. I rode 1,800 miles total last year, but my biggest accomplishment was a 168-mile ride in two days—a fund-raiser for multiple sclerosis. It was a challenging ride, and I was tired afterward. But I felt so strong and happy to be able to complete something that intense.

For me, riding is the key to maintaining my weight. When I exercise regularly, I don't seem to be as hungry. In fact, I've lost another 20 pounds or so; now I'm down to about 130. And I look great in my bike tights.

TAKE-AWAY: Join up

Whether it's a biking group, a hiking club, or a recreational softball league, exercising with a group of people offers many benefits—built-in opportunities for exercise, a social element, a sense of accountability, and a feeling of community.

Praying for Help

Jane, 52, New York, nurse

In August 2001 my sister got married, and I was her matron of honor. Later, when I saw the pictures from the wedding, I was absolutely horrified. I just cried because I couldn't believe I looked like that. And the video—*Oh my gosh!*—the video was even worse. It made me feel so depressed. I thought, "I don't want to live like this; I hate the way I look." I was carrying 282 pounds, and I'm 5 feet 4 inches.

So while I was crying, I got down on my knees and prayed. I said, "God, I can't do this on my own. I need you to help me." I had prayed for help before, but this time I gave it over to God. I acknowledged that I couldn't do it on my own.

My dad, who passed away when I was seventeen, really instilled the importance of faith in me. My husband and I have been part of a wonderful church for the last twenty years, and, in addition to our two grown kids, our congregation is like our family, so praying was nothing new for me. But this prayer was different. It was a desperate plea for help.

I've battled my weight my whole life. I went on my first diet when I was nine years old, and I've tried just about everything that's come along since then—the grapefruit diet, high-protein diets, liquid diets, even Fen-Phen, the drug combination that was taken off the market in 1997 because it caused heart valve problems in some people. I'd lose 5 or 10 pounds, then gain 20, lose 20, and gain 40. Even though my weight-loss attempts were a losing battle, hardly a day has gone by that I haven't worried about my weight or tried to watch what I eat.

I was never one of those people who overate regularly. Sure, I overate at times and I ate fattening foods—I love ice cream—but I also have a terrible metabolism. It's not an excuse. It's reality. I'd eat the same slice of cake that everyone else ate, but it would make me gain weight. It was enormously frustrating. In 1999, I was diagnosed with an underactive thyroid, which can cause a slow metabolism, and I went on medication to increase my thyroid function. That helped a little, in that I didn't seem to gain weight quite as easily after that. But by then I was so heavy it didn't make much difference.

I tried to convince myself that being fat was okay—some people are just heavier than others—but in my heart I knew I could never be happy as a fat person. I'd cry when I couldn't find things to wear and I hated to go shopping. I never looked at my body in the mirror, because I didn't want to see how big I was. I'm a nurse and I am the vice president of my company's home-care division. I felt as if I was in control of my life and successful in every aspect except for my weight. It was awful.

After seeing the pictures from the wedding and asking for God's help, I joined Weight Watchers on September 8, 2001. My goal was to get down to 155 pounds. A part of me didn't believe I would ever get there because I'd failed so many times before. But I developed a routine that I still do to this day: I started to get up at four thirty in the morning for quiet time—Bible reading and prayer. I'd say verse 13 of Philippians, chapter 4: "I can do all things through Him who strengthens me." Then I'd go for a fast two-mile walk. I always hated exercise—hated thinking about it, hated doing it. But I made up my mind that I was going to do everything I could to make this effort work.

"I needed to learn to accept setbacks and to keep believing in myself through them. I had many, many bad days after that, but because I saw them as lessons, they fueled my determination."

I wish I could say the weight loss was easy, but it wasn't. There were lots of upsetting setbacks. I remember going to a meeting after what I thought was a really good week, and the scale had me up 4 pounds. I was so upset, I couldn't stay at the meeting. At that point, I still had more than 100 pounds to lose, and I thought, "I'll never get there at this rate. I'll be 100 years old by the time I reach goal." When I got home, I went into my bedroom and got on my knees. I said,

"Okay, God. I'm really feeling discouraged. I need help." And then it came to me that God was trying to teach me a lesson. I needed to learn to accept setbacks and to keep believing in myself through them. I had many, many bad days after that, but because I saw them as lessons, they fueled my determination. When I'd gain a pound or two, I'd tell myself, "I'm not going to let this defeat me."

One day in the fall of 2005 I went out for my daily morning walk, and as I was striding along I had an unbelievable epiphany: I was enjoying it. Not only did I like walking, but I felt really good. I was eating healthy food and I liked it. The compulsion to eat foods that made me fat was just gone. It may sound hokey, but I think God took it away because every time I felt as if I was losing control, I would say that verse from Philippians, and a sense of peace would come over me. In any case, during that walk I realized that I was cured, healed. Somehow I just knew that this time—for the first time ever—the weight loss was going to stick. And I knew it was because God was helping me.

I reached my initial goal in February 2006, then lost another 22 pounds by July. I've weighed 133 pounds ever since. Recently at work I heard someone describe me as "the tiny little woman over there." I thought, "What? They can't possibly be talking about me." But they were. When I think about the last six years, I realize it hasn't been so much a weight-loss journey as a journey of faith. I'm proud of myself and proud of my effort. But without God's help, I wouldn't be wearing a size 6 today.

TAKE-AWAY: Have faith

When you face setbacks or obstacles in your weight-loss plan or you feel your motivation beginning to wane, rely on your faith in yourself or a higher power to help you pull through.

Getting Healthy in Mind, Body, and Spirit

Kristin, 41, California, exercise instructor

I never had to worry about my weight until I was in my mid-to-late twenties. After I got married, I started to have kids. After the first one, the pregnancy weight stayed with me. After having the second child, I didn't lose the weight, and after the third child, I never lost the weight. I knew I was overweight, but I just sort of ignored it, even though my husband complained a lot.

When we first got married, I slept in the nude. As I gained weight, I stopped sleeping in the nude, and I never wanted to take off my clothes in front of my husband. Between pregnancies, I just wasn't interested in dieting or exercising. I ate whatever I wanted and how much I wanted. I quit caring how I looked or how I felt because I was so busy. Every time I went to the doctor for an appointment, I would say, "Don't tell me how much I weigh," and I wouldn't look. Not knowing how much I weighed made it easy for me to ignore it.

I didn't get on the scale until my gardener asked whether I was pregnant again.

When I finally looked at the scale, I thought, "My goodness. I'm really heavy!" I was up to 190 pounds—I'm 5 feet 3 inches so that felt like a lot.

I started to take step aerobics classes twice a week, but I realized that the exercise wasn't working by itself so I decided to try Weight Watchers. I found out I could follow the plan online and I saw how easy it was, which made me decide to try it. When I began in January 2004, I was shocked to realize how much I was eating—I was probably eating three times as much as I should have been! My husband used to say, "You're eating as much as I'm eating." My husband is 6 feet 1 inch—really, I had no business eating six slices of pizza along with him! So I started to plan what I was going to eat the entire day.

Along the way, I really have changed my eating habits. With pizza, instead of ordering a regular crust, I'll order a thin-crust pizza with veggies and a lighter sauce and less cheese. I don't use mayo or butter anymore. My salad dressings are all low-fat or nonfat. When I eat meat, I look for less-fatty cuts, and I don't eat bacon anymore. When I eat cheese, I always eat a low-fat cheese. We eat salads several nights a week, and I eat lots of vegetables—I love veggies.

It took me eight months to lose 58 pounds. That first week I lost 4 pounds. I knew rationally that a lot of it was water weight, but it made me want to try harder. Because I was enjoying the exercise classes, I added more classes. Once I learned that I could eat more food if I did more exercise, I was like, "Oh, let me exercise more!" Slowly but surely, I was exercising six days a week—and it was for fun. I enjoyed the step classes and the body-sculpting classes. Then I got up to doing about two hours of classes per day. I did a couple of personal training sessions and started lifting weights. Next, I moved to another gym and started to do Pilates and Spinning classes and Tae Bo and kickboxing classes. After that, I started to run half-marathons in 2006.

> "With pizza, instead of ordering a regular crust, I'll order a thin-crust pizza with veggies and a lighter sauce and less cheese. I don't use mayo or butter anymore. My salad dressings are all low-fat or nonfat."

I got totally hooked on exercise and fitness. I never thought I could have fun exercising, but I did. As I kept losing weight, my body got stronger and more toned, and I started to feel healthy in mind, body, and spirit. I became a group exercise instructor and a mat Pilates instructor because I want to motivate other people, to give them the enjoyment that I get out of it. I'd like to inspire them to change their lives.

After losing weight, I started to love my abs. At first, I had a big fold of skin from my abdomen, and I ended up getting a tummy tuck in February 2006, which gave me a flat stomach. Since I started doing Pilates, I have noticed a definite change in my abs. Now you can actually see the shape of my muscles underneath the skin.

I went from skinny and unhealthy to fat and unhealthy to slim and fit. I think I'm at a place where I'm happy with the way I look. I feel confident. I feel sexy. I'm forty-one and I look better than I've ever looked. My body is by no means perfect, but it's perfect to me because I'm fit and I'm healthy and I know it.

TAKE-AWAY: Keep an exercise journal

Make a note of what you did and how the exercise felt, then review your progress regularly—and you'll have a steady source of inspiration to keep up the good workouts.

Consider What You Can Control in Your Life

When life throws a curve ball or a catastrophe hits, you may not be able to control the situation, but you can control your response to it and your behavior, including your eating and exercise habits. Write down several challenges you've recently confronted and how you dealt with them.

_____

_____

_____

_____

_____

_____

_____

_____

_____

_____

_____

CHAPTER 7

Seeking
Good Health

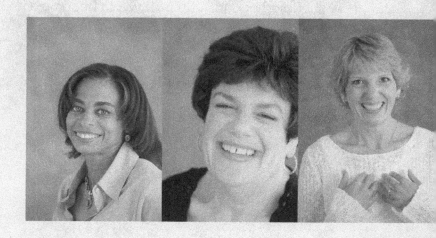

There's nothing like a health scare to inspire a person to clean up his or her act. The men and the women featured in this chapter recount how their excess weight affected their overall health, as well as how their wish to enter the next phase of life spurred them to take action. After reading their stories, you'll learn how your weight could affect your current or future health—and how shedding pounds can help you to become a healthier you.

Saving My Heart

Darla, 44, California, vice chancellor of a university

I woke up one Sunday morning four years ago feeling like I couldn't breathe. I thought I had really bad asthma all of a sudden. I also had a lot of swelling in my ankles. I had no idea why.

I *had* noticed some shortness of breath while walking upstairs at work and I was unable to do my normal walking around, but it was nothing severe. And I'd had a respiratory virus for a couple of months that I couldn't shake, but the symptoms were very slight. It's true I was tired, burned out, not taking care of myself. But that's because I had a lot on my plate. Like many women, I pushed it to the limit, 'til I was exhausted. At thirty-nine, I was a PhD student, I worked full time, and I was married with two children. Anyway, I'd had a physical six months earlier and gotten a clean bill of health.

I called my sister-in-law, who's a physician, and described my symptoms. She said, "I don't want to scare you, but you really should get to the emergency room. It could be really serious."

The ER nurse said, "I bet anything you have a heart virus because those were my symptoms, and they had to carry me out of here on a stretcher."

They did a bunch of tests, and many hours later, my heart barely beating, they discovered that she was right. My doctor's best guess was that I had had that respiratory virus for a long time. Viruses can jump from organ to organ, and it seems that a very invasive virus jumped from my lungs to my heart. It caused my heart to swell, which slowed down its beating.

I was in the hospital for five days. The diagnosis was heart failure. Here, I'd never taken more than an aspirin, and all of a sudden I was faced with taking seven or eight medications a day, to strengthen my heart and regulate its beat and pumping—possibly for the rest of my life! And if the meds didn't work, it was likely that I would need a heart transplant. My head was spinning!

At that point, I made up my mind that I needed to make some lifestyle changes. One was my weight. I weighed around 240 pounds, and the medications soon sent me up to 251. I admit that my weight's always been a struggle. Despite being athletic, I've always been a bigger person. I knew that if I could get some of this weight off, it would probably help my heart.

I joined Weight Watchers and for the first time in my life started to really take care of myself. I couldn't exercise intensely, but I could walk. I lost about 30 pounds. I've been at my current weight of 222 for a while and am getting ready to gear up again. I try to do it 20 or 30 pounds at a time. I have to take breaks because it's exhausting. Even though 222 sounds high, I exercise and eat healthy. Every pound I lose lightens the burden on my heart. That's a good motivator.

"I'm pretty aggressive with exercise. I work out seven days a week for about an hour, a mix of weight lifting and cardio. I have double motivation: every time I work out, I'm strengthening my heart as well as helping myself to lose weight."

I'll take medications for the rest of my life, no matter how much weight I lose. That said, by exercising and losing some weight, I was able to go off one of them, a diuretic. It made me go to the bathroom all day long, so it was great to get to stop.

I'm pretty aggressive with exercise. I work out seven days a week for about an hour, a mix of weight lifting and cardio. I have double motivation: every time I work out, I'm strengthening my heart as well as helping myself to lose weight.

Dropping 30 pounds is one of the things I'm most proud of in my life. It was probably harder than getting my PhD. My weight loss has affected my kids positively, too. Claire, my fourteen-year-old, started to model what I eat and as a result has dropped about fifteen pounds, as her pediatrician had wanted her to do. Now she is very fit and joins me in my workouts almost daily.

My eleven-year-old, Annie, and I are a mother-daughter team of spokespeople for the American Heart Association. Ann was born with a heart defect and had heart surgery when she was four. We share our stories at dinners and other events in the area. She's noticed a difference in my weight, too. Recently, she said, "Gosh, Mommy, your stomach doesn't touch the steering wheel anymore!"

Most women don't realize until it's too late that heart problems kill more women than all the cancers combined. Typically, heart disease has been considered a man's disease. There's a lot of detection with men's heart problems but not with women's.

I try to look at this whole episode as positive: now I really have to take care of myself; I don't have a choice. In a situation where I originally felt very powerless, losing weight and exercising have empowered me. When you're sitting in a hospital bed wondering how the hell you got there, it's important to be able to hold on to that. I probably have another 50 pounds 'til I hit my goal, but I'm going to do it.

My weight loss and better exercise plan have had another positive result: my heart function has improved a lot—I'm now up in the low normal range. It's a small miracle.

TAKE-AWAY: Set a 10 percent milestone
If you have a lot to lose, instead of setting your sights on achieving your ultimate goal, which can feel overwhelming, aim to lose 10 percent of your weight at a time.

Looking toward the Future

Michele, 38, New York, desktop publisher

Right after my thirtieth birthday, I was walking to the train one morning and it dawned on me: My back is aching. I'm sore. It just isn't healthy for my body to carry this much weight. That was what made me think, "I need to do something about this." I weighed about 315 pounds.

After I turned thirty, I did that whole taking-stock thing, and I realized that I want to be healthier at forty than I was at thirty. I went to my doctor, and she recommended that I lose weight. I didn't say, "I need to be at this number"; it was more like, "I need to control my portions, get more fruits and vegetables, make better decisions." I'm lucky that I've always had an hourglass figure. People never, ever thought I was as heavy as I was because I still had curves. It was really about my health.

It was also about seeing ahead into the future and thinking, "I don't want to have health troubles down the road." My dad had emphysema and had to use an oxygen tank. My mom was heavy and developed diabetes. All the things she struggled with, I could see that in my future. Also, my husband and I have been married about four years, and we want to have kids so that was a factor, too. I want to be able to run around and play with them and enjoy them.

When I started to lose weight, I did try to keep in mind that I'd had thirty years of poor eating and lack of exercise. Basically, I was a thirty-year-old geek. I do computer stuff and have a lot of sedentary hobbies. I decided that, first, I wanted to get my eating in check. A lot of times, if I went overboard with my eating, I'd sit down and write about why. Sometimes something was bothering me, so I'd have to say to myself, "Why do I want this particular food?" Now I'm a lot more thoughtful about what I eat and why I'm eating it.

Then, as I started to lose weight, I tried some activities. I took baby steps, then got more active. Now, at the gym, I take a belly dancing class that I love. I also do yoga, and I love that because there's that whole connecting with the body and making sure everything's in line and calming down. That's become more important as I get older.

As part of my taking stock, I really needed to focus on what was important. I found a suggestion early on of putting together a top-ten list of the reasons you want to lose weight. Some of my top reasons are to be healthy, which is simple to say, harder to do; to stop food from controlling me and to learn to control it; and to be able to enjoy physical activities without having to wonder whether I can keep up with them. To stay motivated, I'll go back and check that. I'll think, "Why did I want to lose?" Then, "Why do I want to maintain it?"

I'm thirty-eight now, and I have reached my goal of 183 pounds. I feel as if I have a lot more energy. I don't have the back pain anymore, and I can do more without getting tired. My husband and I go up to the Adirondack Mountains, and we can do day hikes now. There's no way I could have done that before—and I really enjoy it. Now I'm usually ahead of him. It's like I'm bookin' ahead, and he's going, "Wait, wait, wait." I'm so much better off than I was at thirty and I'm better prepared to deal with the next challenge—forty.

> "Some of my top reasons to lose weight are to be healthy, which is simple to say, harder to do; to stop food from controlling me and to learn to control it; and to be able to enjoy physical activities without having to wonder whether I can keep up with them."

TAKE-AWAY: Think hard about why you want to lose weight

If you jot down a list of your primary reasons for wanting to slim down, you'll have a handy source of inspiration when your motivation begins to flag.

Gaining a Positive Attitude
with Cancer

Donna, 52, Texas, governmental policy adviser

I would never have chosen to have breast cancer, of course, but it gave me a better perspective. It gave me more appreciation for life. It also inspired me to lose weight.

My breast cancer was diagnosed on March 9, 1999. It had spread to four of my lymph nodes. I had a mastectomy, six months of chemo, thirty-eight radiation treatments, and breast reconstruction. My thyroid stopped functioning correctly because of the radiation, which made me heavier than I had ever been. Ever since puberty, I have been overweight, but after the radiation treatments, I put on another 30 pounds.

But I got through the cancer treatments and went back to work as a policy adviser for the governor's office, where I write legislation and work with legislators. During the legislative session, it can be a little crazy. For a while, I hadn't done anything about losing the weight. Then, in July 2001, a friend at work came up and asked me whether I wanted to join Weight Watchers At Work. I was one of the heaviest people in the office and I was her supervisor. I thought, "Okay, I won't be a very good role model if I don't do this."

I skipped the first two meetings because I was pretty sure I weighed over 200 at that point and I didn't want to weigh in at over 200. So I waited a couple of weeks and cut down on what I was eating. At my first weigh-in, I was 198. My goal at that point was to get down to 141 because I'm just 5 feet 3 inches.

When I started, what I really wanted was to feel better. I looked terrible and I felt terrible. I knew losing weight would make me healthier—and I wanted to be around for a long time. When I was diagnosed with breast cancer, my sons, Johnny and Cote, were just eight and sixteen.

I followed the program and I began running. A year later, I had lost about 48 pounds—I was down to 150, not quite to my goal. But then I began what became a terrible plateau. The scale just did not move. Around November 2002, I thought, "I am just going to be happy at 150." I stopped attending meetings, but I still ate healthy, and I still exercised, too. In fact, in June 2003, I ran in Grandma's Marathon in Duluth, Minnesota.

In the fall of 2004, I heard a lecture by a breast cancer doctor at the breast cancer resource center I go to. She said that being at your ideal weight can reduce your risk of breast cancer recurrence. I thought, "This is craziness. I need to lose the rest of this weight to get down to my ideal weight."

So after more than two years of not going to Weight Watchers meetings, I went back in December 2004. I remember the leader, Julie, saying to me and the new people, "You must be really committed if you are joining between Thanksgiving and Christmas."

I set 141 as my goal and I hit it a month later, on January 29, 2005. It was very emotional for me. Decreasing my odds of recurrence is what drove me. I wanted to be around for my sons, who are now seventeen and twenty-five, when they grow up. I know they need me. My older son is autistic. He now lives in a group home for adults with disabilities that is near our house, but he comes back home just about every other weekend. I'm his lifeline, the person he depends on.

"Fighting the cancer successfully and losing the weight had everything to do with my positive attitude. I realized that life is short and you need to live every moment. When I look back on my life, I don't want to say, 'Gosh, I've had a lot of really good meals.'"

After I hit 141 pounds, I tried to maintain that. It was when the legislature was in session so it was a very stressful time and I just kept losing. By June 2005, I had gotten down to 130 pounds—in all, I had lost 68 pounds. I now wear a size 4, and sometimes even a size 2. I used to be a size 18 or 20.

I am not the least bit concerned about putting this weight back on. Early on, I decided that I wouldn't do anything to lose this weight that I was not willing to do the rest of my life. It's not a diet; it's a healthy way to eat.

Fighting the cancer successfully and losing the weight had everything to do with my positive attitude. I realized that life is short and you need to live every moment. If you spend time with bitterness, it takes away from your opportunities for having all the good things in life. The other thing that has helped me tremendously is the realization that food is not the be-all and end-all. When I look back on my life, I don't want to say, "Gosh, I've had a lot of really good meals." I want to say, "I had so many good friends, such a good family, and such a blessed life."

TAKE-AWAY: Start a gratitude diary

Each day, jot down three to five things you're grateful for in your life in a special diary. When your spirits flag or you're in the midst of an especially aggravating day, paging through your diary can bolster your mood and your resolve to stay on track with your goals.

Taking the Pressure
off Myself

Trudie, 44, Georgia, Weight Watchers leader

On a Sunday afternoon in August 2003, I had a horrible headache that sent me to the emergency room. I was very overweight, and I'd been struggling with bad headaches and not feeling good for a while. Back then, I was always drinking sodas and coffee and eating candy so I honestly believed that I was having caffeine-withdrawal headaches and needed more caffeine. That day, I felt lightheaded and dizzy and my headache would not go away, even after I had lain down, had coffee, and taken aspirin. I just did not want to get up and do anything, which was not normal for me. My husband finally said, "We're going to get this checked out," so we went to the hospital.

As my husband, my two children, and I sat in the waiting room in the ER, I asked my husband whether he would get me a soda and a candy bar because maybe they would help me feel better. He did, and I drank and ate them while we waited. When they finally checked me, they told me that my blood pressure was more than 200/140 mm Hg—at stroke level! It had been a little high before, but I was shocked that it was as high as it was. The doctor told me that all of my symptoms—my headaches, the lightheadedness, feeling lethargic—were related to my blood pressure being so high and that I needed to get on medication.

Then it all came flooding back to me. I thought, "Oh my gosh! This was my mom." She had high blood pressure and died from a heart attack at fifty-two. Here I was having extreme high blood pressure, and I knew what the results were—that you could die from a heart attack or a stroke. Suddenly, I saw myself in her.

The doctor also vaguely mentioned, almost as a side note, that a proper diet, exercise, and losing weight would help. But he said it almost like, "This is something we have to say as doctors, but nobody ever really does it." At that point, my weight was about 207, and I'm 5 feet 2 inches.

I was never a small person—my weight was always pretty much around 140 or 150—but it crept up little by little. Before I got married, I went on a liquid diet, lost 30 pounds, and was a small bride like I dreamed of being. I'm sure that before the honeymoon was over, I couldn't have fit into my wedding dress again. On the honeymoon, I started eating again for the first time after being on that liquid diet—and I never stopped after that. After having two children, I joined one of the quick weight-loss centers. Then I did the diet where the meals were sent to my home. Other times, I went and had shots or took pills that made my heart beat really fast.

But that day at the emergency room just woke me up. I lost 5 pounds on my own, then decided to sign up for Weight Watchers. When I found out that the recommended weight loss was half a pound to 2 pounds per week, that was discouraging because I felt like I was in an emergency-type situation and that was going to take too long. I thought, "I need to lose 30 pounds in thirty days!" So I was not sitting there as an eager member. But because I had tried everything else, I thought I would give it a chance and see how it went.

The amazing thing is, it wasn't all that hard for me to get results early on. Initially, I ate some of the same things I used to eat, but when I started to lose weight, I said, "Well, what if I eat even better? What if I cut out sodas, what would happen?" So I stopped keeping soda and juice in the house. I stopped having a lot of snacks in the house. We don't have as much processed food as we used to, and we have more vegetables and fruit. We stopped eating while watching TV, which we always used to do. Now I think, "Don't put those two together—either eat or watch TV—because when you eat while watching TV, it becomes mindless eating." Little by little, I just kept making small changes that eventually became a healthy eating process. But it all started from baby steps.

And I was feeling better! I used to get out of breath coming up the steps. My back used to hurt. My knees hurt. Even before I started to look better, I began to feel better and that was probably the best motivator. Once I lost weight, I wasn't huffing and puffing anymore. My knees didn't hurt. I didn't feel tired all the time the way I used to. My headaches stopped. Then I got my own blood pressure monitor, started to check it at home, and it consistently kept going down.

Another thing that kept me motivated was my children. My daughter was my little imitator; she copied everything that I did. She wanted to put on my shoes and jewelry, and she ate with me. I realized that I needed to set the best example I could for her so she wouldn't struggle with these issues. I was twenty-one when my mom passed, and I felt like that was still very young. I

"Even before I started to look better, I began to feel better and that was probably the best motivator.

thought, "I don't want to leave my daughter a young woman without her mom if I can help it." I felt a nudging strength that I had to do better for her and for my family.

At one point, my weight loss slowed down so I increased my exercise. At first, I walked three days a week for twenty minutes, which was a major, big deal for me because I don't come from an active background. Now I work out four to five times a week, for thirty to sixty minutes. I walk on my treadmill, and I follow the basic training or strength-training shows on Fit TV.

Over fourteen months, I lost 72 pounds, and I'm down to 130. I try to stay within a 5-pound range max because I think I can handle 5 pounds, but once it goes beyond that, it's so much harder. I weigh myself every day to make sure I'm within the range that's workable for me. My blood pressure is normal now—without medication—but it will go up if I don't exercise. Now I try to never go more than two days without exercise so that my blood pressure stays under control. It's my limit.

A while ago, I realized how much thinner I really am when my husband and I saw someone we hadn't seen in two years. He kind of pulled my husband aside and asked whether we'd broken up. My husband said, "No, that's her." The man looked at me and was like, "Oh my God! You look great!" I was shocked because I didn't think I looked unrecognizable, but my husband was a little offended. He was like, "I can't believe you didn't know it was her!"

In February 2007, we renewed our vows after sixteen years of marriage. And the wedding dress I wore the second time was better and I felt prettier than I did the first time. I felt better about my body at forty-three than I had when I got married in my twenties.

TAKE-AWAY: Don't eat while watching TV

If you do, eating becomes mindless, and before you know it, you can have eaten too much—without even really enjoying, or truly noticing, what you've consumed.

Losing Weight
to Save My Life

Peter, 39, Georgia, founder of a nonprofit to raise awareness and
money for organ transplants

My kidneys never developed properly, and by 1983, when I was fourteen, I had to have a kidney transplant. I'd always been skinny and underweight, and I went in for that first surgery weighing just 90 pounds. For a year before that, I'd drunk protein drinks to boost my weight, which didn't work. But they had to do the surgery anyway. That first kidney came from my mom and lasted sixteen years.

After the transplant, I went from 90 pounds to 120 in a month, due to the steroids I took to prevent organ rejection. I was on a strict diet: low protein, low carbs, low sodium, because any extra weight was stress on my body. But I put on weight anyway.

It was an ongoing living hell. I suddenly had to avoid gaining weight, and everything I ate was bland, like popcorn with nothing on it. I was deprived of food that I wanted, especially fast food, and people made fun of me. Transplant patients often have round faces. It's called a moon face. I looked like the Stay Puft Marshmallow Man from *Ghostbusters*. My nickname in my family—my brother gave it to me—was the Pillsbury Doughboy. That still stays with me when I get big, which is a great motivation to lose weight.

The first two or three years after my transplant, I was very self-conscious. It was tough to go into a store and say, "I need a pair of jeans. By the way, I need *huskies*." I was only 5 feet tall and not very energetic. Before the surgery, I'd always been energetic.

Gradually, I got more active because my weight made me self-conscious, and being active helped me to get my strength and energy back. Then, when I was sixteen, I learned to water-ski. It drove my doctors and my mom crazy—they worried that I'd fall and damage my kidneys. I was on the tennis team. My weight got down to about

110. Not only did I become active, I was more conscious about what I ate: bran rather than sugared cereals, eggs without bacon.

But as I got into my twenties, my weight moved up—to 130 pounds. My doctors were thrilled, but I said, "No, I can't gain weight! I'm too fat!" The doctors said, "No, Peter, you need to stay at 125. You're fine where you are."

But I really didn't pay attention. I started jogging and white-water kayaking, and I got down to 119. It was a great time for me. Party every day! I put on weight; I lost weight. I ignored my health problems—really, I denied that I had any problems. Everything was going great, weight-wise and health-wise, and I was about to graduate from culinary school.

Then one day, I went to see my doctor. He said, "I don't like the way the blood test came back for your second kidney." I took it again the next day, and he put me right in the hospital for a biopsy. I've never before seen a doctor shed tears. I looked at him and said, "I've lost my kidney."

My second kidney came from my aunt, my mom's sister, in December 2004. After that transplant, my weight went up to about 140. I tried to exercise, but other medical problems came up and it was a real struggle.

I maxed out with my weight in December 2006 at 184 pounds—again, largely because of the steroids and inactivity. I was miserable. I couldn't walk for fifteen minutes without sitting down and feeling as if I was hyperventilating. I was depressed so I ran to my comfort foods: peanut butter, graham crackers, milk, and bananas.

I remember the day I decided to go to Weight Watchers. I bent down to tie my shoes and I couldn't breathe. I thought, "I've always been healthy. I've run. I've been a white-water kayaker. I've backpacked. And now I can't bend over to tie my shoes?!" I was so angry with myself. I went into losing weight as if it were life or death. I had to do it to save myself, to feel good about myself.

Besides starting the program, I began to exercise. I couldn't walk fifteen minutes without taking breaks, so fifteen minutes would take me twenty-five minutes. I did it every day.

I started cycling when I couldn't walk or run anymore because of the steroids and the previous running injuries. Within just a few weeks, I built up on the stationary bike to three and a half hours a day, with a five-minute break every hour.

And that's when I thought about riding across America for transplant awareness and donor education. I've been training on the road, and I've had two good wrecks! I formed a nonprofit organization, Team Green Cycle, and we decided that I would start by biking all over Georgia, eighteen hundred miles in four and a half weeks for the first try in October 2007. Half of the money raised will go to the Georgia Transplant Foundation and the National Kidney Foundation, and a part will come back to Team Green.

> "I started cycling when I couldn't walk or run anymore because of the steroids and the previous running injuries. Within just a few weeks, I built up on the stationary bike to three and a half hours a day, with a five-minute break every hour."

I've made my lifetime goal of 150, and now I'm at 148. My doctors don't want me below 150 with all the cycling and training I'm doing. I can finally say I like my calves: I looked at my legs a few weeks ago, and I thought my calves were swollen. Then, it dawned on me that since I've been cycling and losing weight, I've got muscle definition. Wow! That's pretty cool to me.

My life has been fuller than I can ever put into words. I'm so blessed. If everything stopped right now, I'd be happy with what I left behind because I feel so fulfilled with everything in my life. And I know it's just going to get better.

TAKE-AWAY: Build up your exercise gradually

Even if you can walk for only five or ten minutes without stopping at first, continue to put one foot in front of the other and take breaks as needed. If you listen to your body's comfort signals and increase your time or distance slowly, you'll be able to condition your heart, lungs, and muscles without risking injury or burnout.

Keeping a Sense
of Humor

Bettyann, 58, New York, retired high school English teacher

Gastric bypass surgery. Those three words changed my life, but not in the way you might think.

In July 2004 I was visiting my doctor to get some blood work done when he scared me straight. "You're going to keep having health problems unless you take off some weight," he said. "I strongly recommend bariatric surgery." It's a surgery that would limit how much I can eat and the calories my body absorbs. He'd been worried about my health for a while. I'd had gallstones, gallbladder surgery, liver problems, and bile duct stones—all because I was overweight. I was fifty-five years old and nearly 300 pounds—a lot for anyone, but I'm only 5 feet 1 inch. He had encouraged me to diet in the past, but I always told him, "Somebody's gotta be fat, doc. It might as well be me. At least, I'm happy."

But deep down I knew that wasn't really true. I was ashamed that I couldn't sit in regular theater seats or vacuum behind the sofa or squeeze through the turnstile at Shea Stadium when the whole family would go see baseball games. But I'd hold my head high as I went through the stadium's door for disabled people. It was humiliating to have to use it because I was heavy, but I didn't have a choice. Still, I thought I was too far gone to lose weight.

But I was taken aback by the idea of surgery. I'd already been sliced and diced every which way, and I hate anesthesia. It makes me hyper for days. I thought, "Am I such a hopeless case that I can't lose weight by myself?" So I decided to show the doctor that I could do it. His nurse suggested I try Weight Watchers. I thought that sounded almost as bad as surgery! I'm not one to weigh or count anything. I'm Italian, and I cook every day. Eggplant parmigiana, steak pizzaiola, lasagna, baked ziti—those recipes are in my blood, and making them is how I show my family how much I love them and want to take care of them.

That's the most important thing in the world to me. But I realized that I had to take care of me. I had a choice: count **POINTS** or have surgery. So I dragged myself to a Saturday meeting.

I was determined to hate it. I sat there with a bad attitude, with my arms crossed, thinking, "There's no way this is going to help me." But my meeting leader won me over. She was funny, and we laughed at each other's jokes. It's been three years now, and we've laughed during every meeting. I mean it. We laugh at how hard it is to stick with it and how there are times when you're so hungry you could eat the linoleum off the floor. And we laugh at our changing bodies. I've lost more than 130 pounds over the last three years, and my legs and arms are skinny as anything, but my middle is like a deflated inner tube. Some people in my place might want to have surgery, but I see it differently. It's a daily reminder of how far I've come— and a warning of what could be again. When I look in the mirror, I say to myself, "You don't ever want to inflate that thing again."

In the spring of 2005, my twenty-six-year-old son, James, and I went to see a Mets game. As we walked up to Shea Stadium, I headed for the disabled door, as usual. But James looked at me and said, "Give it a try, Mom," and steered me toward the turnstile. For a moment, I felt panicky because I thought I was still way too big. But I pushed right through it. I burst into tears, and James swept me up in a big bear hug.

> "I was determined to hate it. I sat there with a bad attitude, with my arms crossed, thinking, 'There's no way this is going to help me.' But my meeting leader won me over. She was funny, and we laughed at each other's jokes."

TAKE-AWAY: Keep your sense of humor

As you navigate the weight-loss journey, try to see the humorous side of things, whether it's marveling at how healthy your new cravings are, how your body is changing, or how you've become hooked on exercise.

Bye-Bye, Diabetes

Robin, 51, Tennessee, personal assistant

I'm a high-energy person. I talk fast and I'm usually crazy-busy. I drive my family a little nuts because when I decide something needs to be done, I have to get it done immediately—like *now*. I home-schooled my two daughters all the way through elementary and high school and helped my husband, a youth minister, with his job. But about ten years ago, when my younger daughter was eleven and my older daughter had just started college, I noticed that I was getting really tired all the time, especially when I ate poorly—which is something I did a lot.

I'm a huge snacker and crazy for sweets. I would sometimes eat a whole box of chocolate-covered caramels or a bag of cookies in one sitting. If I was in the mood for a candy bar, I might eat three. Afterward, I'd feel so tired I often had to take a nap. It was almost as if I went into a coma. I remember one time we went out to dinner with some friends and I ate a really sweet, rich dessert. We came back to our house afterward to talk, and I fell asleep on the sofa right in front of our guests!

I was also thirsty all the time—this sort of unreal thirst that I couldn't ever satisfy. And I was grouchy. I told my gynecologist about the symptoms, and she tested me for type 2 diabetes. I wasn't surprised when the test came back positive because I was way overweight. I weighed 236 pounds, and my doctor had been warning me that I was at risk for diabetes. But I just couldn't lose weight. And my health had finally deteriorated as a result.

I started taking Glucophage pills twice a day to control my blood sugar. I felt pretty low about that. I knew I was responsible for what was happening with my health, but I just couldn't seem to control my eating. I felt even worse when my husband changed jobs and his new health insurance wouldn't cover me. Here I was without coverage, and it was all my fault.

I took the medicine religiously every day, but it became less and less effective at controlling my blood sugar, and my doctor said that if we couldn't find a way to get it under control with pills, I'd have to start giving myself insulin injections. That really scared me. I didn't want to have to live that way for the rest of my life.

Finally, in the fall of 2005, I went with a friend for a get-away week-end. She had just lost weight on Weight Watchers, and all weekend I watched the way she ate. I was amazed at how much food she ate—and she had great sweet snacks, too. I went home and signed up right away.

It wasn't easy to change my eating habits, but I gradually developed a strategy that works for me. At mealtime I try to fill up by eating as many vegetables as I can because I like to feel full. If I'm walking around hungry, I'm way more likely to eat something I shouldn't. So I'll make a big salad or broth soup with cabbage and carrots and onions and green beans. I'll eat that way all day so I can have three or four 100-calorie snacks at night when I'm spending time with the family, reading, or watching TV. That's when I'm most vulnerable to overeating. I'll have fat-free pudding or popcorn or mini cupcakes or a granola bar. I keep a variety of snacks on hand so that I don't get bored with any one thing.

"I'll make a big salad or broth soup with cabbage and carrots and onions and green beans. I'll eat that way all day so I can have three or four 100-calorie snacks at night when I'm spending time with the family, reading, or watching TV."

After I began eating that way, the weight really started to come off—and I was able to cut back on my medication. Then, in April 2006, I went to my doctor and he gave me amazing news. I no longer had diabetes; my blood sugar was now normal, even without medication. I kept his note. It said: "Keep up the good work with continued diet, exercise, and weight loss. It's as if you had never been diabetic." That was just the best feeling. It was like starting a new life because I realized that as long as I kept my weight under control, I didn't need to worry as much about my health.

On November 22, the day before my fiftieth birthday, I reached my goal weight of 164 pounds. My husband and I have been able to get the same health insurance again, and I feel great physically. I do the elliptical machine at the gym for thirty minutes five days a week, and I have plenty of energy to get through the day. I never have that lethargic feeling after I eat anymore.

After my younger daughter left home, I became a personal assistant to a woman who owns a day spa, and I'm always on the go. I shop for her and run all her errands. I'm going, going, going all the time—but thanks to my new diet, my energy is never gone.

TAKE-AWAY: Budget for splurges

If you enjoy snacking in the evening, at the movies, or any other time, you don't have to give up these pleasurable experiences if you plan for them ahead of time.

Participate in Physical Activities You Used to Love

Think about what forms of movement you truly enjoyed in your childhood: jumping rope, playing touch football, dancing, ice-skating. Seek out opportunities to reconnect to your former self. What are the words you would use to describe how you want to feel after engaging in activity?

_____

_____

_____

_____

_____

_____

_____

_____

_____

_____

_____

_____

_____

_____

CHAPTER 8

A Guy Thing

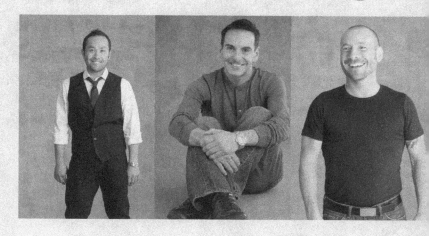

As with many things in life, when it comes to weight-related matters, there's often a gender gap. Traditionally, what inspired men to lose weight has been a personal health scare or the death of a friend. Yet more men than ever are choosing to lose weight to look and feel better—on the job and at home. In this chapter, you'll hear from men who've struggled with their weight at various stages of their lives and found ways to win the battle by cleaning up their eating habits and beefing up their exercise regimens. Their stories about where they went wrong, how they came to view themselves, and what they did to change their ways will inspire men and women alike as you embark on your get-healthy journey to a thinner you.

Healthy = Happy

Ron Darling, 47, New York, TV baseball analyst covering the Mets; former Mets pitcher

I'm nearing my fiftieth birthday, and I decided that I needed to find an avenue to start living healthier. I wanted to get back to my playing weight because I've put on more than 20 pounds since my pitching days. I also want to be more active with my kids—and be around longer for them. So I started doing Weight Watchers Online for Men while my friends and family do it with me.

For me, the biggest challenge is eating on the road. I'm always traveling for my gig as a broadcaster for the Mets, so I'm in and out of airports for the better part of six months. That means I needed to change the way I choose food, particularly on planes and in airports. Being on the road, I don't always have healthy food options so I've learned how to make better choices wherever I am. Instead of eating ballpark food when I'm covering a game, I'll get a turkey sandwich. After I'm done with work at midnight, I like to have a couple of drinks and just chill. But instead of having mixed drinks or a cheeseburger, which I've found not to be worth the **POINTS**, I'll have a couple of light beers and a shrimp cocktail.

I don't look at food the same way anymore. I still love eating, but now I'm much more aware of what goes into my mouth. As a player, I used to eat up to 5,000 calories a day, but I didn't have to think about it because I'd just work it off the next day.

I never consciously thought about what I was eating when I was eating it. It probably had something to do with the fact that as a kid, I was always taught to clean my plate. I'm still cleaning my plate: I just don't have as much on it to begin with now that I've learned about portion control. I don't have to have a twenty-ounce steak; now I'm happy with half of that. When my wife and I go out to dinner, we'll have an appetizer and we'll share an entrée—and I still feel plenty full. The biggest change I made to my lifestyle is eating breakfast. Everyone told me it was important, but I have always hated breakfast food; now I'll at least have a bowl of oatmeal.

My weight-loss mantra is "Move forward every day." I do some kind of exercise every day: walking on the treadmill for an hour, lifting weights, or playing golf or basketball when I can. These days, I try to only play at places where I can walk instead of taking a cart; I've walked five to seven miles, depending on the course.

Weight loss is a lot like baseball: you have to be in it for the long haul. The guys who are really good at it are the ones who pay attention to the details and work hard every day. It's the same with weight loss. If you have a bad day, the key is not to beat yourself up but to play through it. There've been times when I've experienced a little lull in my weight loss, and it can definitely be discouraging. What I try to do is remind myself that I spent twenty years putting on the extra weight, and I can't expect it to come off quickly.

> "Weight loss is a lot like baseball: you have to be in it for the long haul. The guys who are really good at it are the ones who pay attention to the details and work hard every day."

I knew I'd reached a turning point when I had to go to the tailor and get my suits refitted. That made me feel pretty darn proud of myself. The guys at work have also noticed a change in the way I look.

While losing weight, I've discovered that the same old competitiveness is still there. I still want to win. I'm already under the playing weight of my last season, and I'm aiming for my weight of 1984. I think I can pull it off.

These days, I feel good. My joints and muscles ache less, my face is thinner, and I've got more energy than my kids, which is a feat in itself. I'm not trying to lose weight to be gaunt or to look like someone else. I'm trying to be healthy. Skinny does not equal happy. Healthy equals happy.

TAKE-AWAY: Don't beat yourself up about bad eating days

If you seriously overindulge on a particular day, look at it as a minor setback and get right back on track with your get-healthy plan at the next meal or the next morning.

Scared Serious

Rolando, 41, New Jersey, beer salesman

We were a fat family. Growing up, we were always encouraged to eat, always encouraged to have seconds. No one ever said, "Don't eat too much," or "You can't have that." My mother said that I wasn't fat, I was healthy. She was my mother so, of course, I believed her. I remember in fourth or fifth grade, someone's mother came to our class. She was thin, and I thought, "She's a mother?! How can she be a mother if she's not overweight?"

The first time I tried to do anything about my weight, I took diet pills. I did lose weight—and gained it back. In college I tried eating just once a day, one very small meal. I lost a lot of weight, but not in a healthy way. Other times, I lost weight because I exercised so much, but the cold weather would come and I'd say that I couldn't bicycle because it was cold.

At my heaviest, I was 272 pounds. I'm 5 feet 8 inches. That first time I joined Weight Watchers, I dropped weight pretty quickly by watching what I ate and exercising every day for an hour at least. In May 2000 I reached my goal. Basically, I did everything by the book.

The problem is, that's all I did. I was living with my sister and didn't have any responsibilities outside of going to work. I didn't appreciate the weight loss because I had done it so fast and unrealistically. I thought, "This is easy!" As soon as I got to my goal, I started to put weight back on.

By January 2005, I had regained most of what I'd lost. I finally decided that I had to do it the right way: to be realistic and make weight loss work with my life. A combination of things convinced me. I got my cholesterol tested, and it was 201. That's not way too high, but it was high enough for someone who has diabetes in the family, as I do. And I hated the way I looked. I'd get out of the shower, look in the mirror, and call myself names like "fat pig."

But the real defining moment came one day at work. I started to get pains in my chest so I went to the emergency room. They had difficulty getting a good read on the MRI because of my weight. I lay there at the hospital for nine hours—many hours longer than if I'd been thin—and I thought, "I could have died." In the end, they didn't even find anything wrong; they chalked it up to stress. But that was it. I said, "This is enough. I can't keep beating myself up. I have to make a change." I didn't want to keep yo-yoing, but I'd never really believed I had to make *real* changes.

Before, I'd been a secret dieter. This time I told everyone—friends, family, coworkers—that I was trying to lose. This helped me to stick with it.

I started slowly and I wrote down everything I was eating. As I got closer to a 10-pound loss, I became a little more serious about eating accurate portions—not just guesstimating—and about squeezing in exercise. After that, weight loss was a little more consistent.

> "Now it's part of my daily routine to get up in the morning, pack my lunch, go to work, go to the gym. Everything's always prepared. I always know in advance what I'm going to eat. Planning and writing things down are the key."

I've stayed within a few pounds of my goal of 162 for a year now—the longest I've ever kept the weight off. Every other time, as soon as I got comfortable, I went back to eating the way I had before. Not this time. Now it's part of my daily routine to get up in the morning, pack my lunch, go to work, go to the gym. Everything's always prepared. I always know in advance what I'm going to eat. For example, if I'd stopped to have lunch instead of bringing it with me, I might have had fast food. Planning and writing things down are the key.

As the pounds dropped, I made it a priority to get exercise in. I didn't want to lose weight and be flabby. I keep my gym bag in the car and go on the way home. I do cardiovascular and strength training, five to six days a week, for ninety minutes.

Sometimes I need motivation to keep eating this way because it can get monotonous. That's when I think about how I felt when I was heavier, or I look at old pictures. I don't want to be that person again. I don't want to feel like I felt or look how I used to look.

Not only do I look like a whole different person, I feel like a different person. I hated having those large clothes, which I've gotten rid of. I was miserable and angry when I was heavier. I'd get upset and take jokes as an attack, even jokes that weren't about weight. Now I feel happy, excited, friendly. I'm more outgoing.

In Costa Rica, on a vacation with people I work with, I went surfing for the first time and tried a zipline, where you fly through the jungle in a harness on a cable between the trees. I wouldn't have done that when I was overweight. We did a jungle tour where we walked up and down hills. My coworkers were sweating and out of breath—and I was fine. I loved it! Seeing them struggling was one more motivator to stay on track. That's a mantra I always say: "Stay on track! Stay on track!"

TAKE-AWAY: Plan your meals

When you plan what you're going to eat ahead of time—by packing a lunch to take to work or preparing dinner in advance—you take the guesswork and spontaneity out of eating when you're ravenous.

Finding the Courage to Change—Twice

Wayne, 64, Arkansas, retired attorney

I've always used the Serenity Prayer to help me get by: "Give me the serenity to accept the things I cannot change, the courage to change the ones I can, and the wisdom to know the difference." I'm a recovering alcoholic, and I learned the prayer when I quit drinking in 1994, but it helps me in all kinds of other situations, too. It might be something trivial, like someone being rude to me in the supermarket or cutting me off in traffic. Or something more major, like a death in the family. It helps me to sort out what is worth getting upset about because I can do something about it and what isn't because I just can't change it. A side effect of quitting drinking was that I started to eat a lot more sweets and I gained a lot of weight—about 120 pounds. I had already been heavy. As it turned out, the Serenity Prayer helped me in this regard, too.

Being fat was one of the things I didn't think I could change in my life, and I'd sort of fooled myself into thinking I was happy the way I was. I'd been fighting obesity since I was in my twenties, but after I got out of the army in the 1960s, it really got bad. I'm 6 feet 6 inches, so I can carry a lot of weight, but not 420 pounds. It caused all sorts of problems in my daily life. I had to ask for a seat-belt extension in airplanes, and I couldn't fit into the seats at all at the ballpark or in concert auditoriums, so I'd have to stand in the back. My wife and I live on a lake, and we have a boat, but you have to go down an incline to get to it. It got so that I didn't want to go on the boat because I knew how hard it was for me to get back up. I'd think long and hard before heading down there because I didn't want to have to go back up for anything.

I thought that being big wasn't my fault. The way I saw it, my wife and I ate all the same foods, and she wasn't fat, so it must be a genes thing. I didn't realize that having one cookie isn't the same as having four or five—I just thought, "Oh, a few more cookies won't hurt me. That second helping of potatoes and gravy, or some more cornbread dressing, or another roll, or a third piece of garlic bread—they can't be that bad." My daddy was big, and I was big. I just assumed that it was my lot in life, and I made up my mind to accept it.

But I guess in the back of my mind I was always looking for some way out of my situation because in 2005, when a friend of mine lost 60 pounds on Weight Watchers, I decided to give it a try. Being so heavy, I saw success right away, and that made me think, "Okay, maybe I was wrong; maybe my obesity is one of the things I *can* change." But I had to be realistic. The chart told me I should weigh 211. Well, I haven't weighed that since I got out of high school. I went to the doctor and he told me that 240 to 245 would be a good weight for me.

> "My meeting leader gradually got me to start thinking instead about what I *could* eat—lots of fruit, popcorn, lean hamburgers, low-fat ice cream, healthy frozen dinners, and one piece of garlic bread, not three."

Losing 200 pounds took more courage than I thought I ever had. It was going to the meetings that gave me the strength to change my habits. As a recovering alcoholic, I know how important it is to be able to sit with people who are in a similar situation and encourage one another. When I first started, I didn't think I could handle planning out all my meals. When you're used to eating anything you want, you think, "God, this is so limiting! How am I going to do it?" And I was afraid of being hungry. When I did a liquid diet back in the 1980s, I remember being so hungry I felt like I'd eat an easy chair if you put salt and pepper on it!

So in the beginning I spent all this time thinking about the things I couldn't eat. But then my meeting leader gradually got me to start thinking instead about what I *could* eat—lots of fruit, popcorn, lean hamburgers, low-fat ice cream, healthy frozen dinners, and one piece of garlic bread, not three. If you'd have asked me to try turnip greens, pickled beets, or a veggie burger a few years ago, I'd have laughed or said, "No way; that's stupid." But now I actually *like* those things. My tastes changed. I took the bowls of dry-roasted peanuts and cookies off the table and forced myself to give up the habit of reaching for a big handful whenever I was bored. And then it just became normal to eat the healthy stuff. I lost 178 pounds, then surprised even myself by keeping on until I weighed about 217.

There's a famous running back for the L.A. Rams who, when someone asked him how he did it, said something like, "I don't know. When I watch films of my plays, I amaze even myself." That's how I feel. When I look at my wife, who weighs 102 pounds, and think that I used to walk around as if I was holding one of her in each hand, I hardly know how I got through life before or how I finally lost the weight. Now I look back on my life and see that I was making all the wrong choices, without knowing I could choose differently. Sure, I wish I'd have learned the truth before, but the past is the past and all I can do is get on with it and enjoy life now. When I see people in the kind of shape I was in, I really feel for them and I wish they had the wisdom I have now. Happiness for me is just being able to live what to other people is a normal life. Like going to a triple-A baseball game in Little Rock and sitting in the normal seats or hiking with my two grown kids or getting scuba certified, then being able to use those skills in the Pacific Ocean in Mexico.

To me, it's pretty extraordinary. These days my nightly routine includes thanking God for giving me the courage to make these things a part of my regular life.

TAKE-AWAY: Let your environment support your goals

Take away the bowls of chips and nuts, get rid of the junk food in your cabinets or pantry, and put a bowl of fresh fruit on the kitchen table. This way, you'll have healthy choices staring you in the face when you're hungry.

Losing Weight Is a Family Affair

Tracy, 44, New Jersey, bus driver

My mother used to say there was no stopping me, that's how active I was as a child. I was into sports, in great shape; I was never heavy. Then in my twenties, I stopped smoking, and I practically went insane with hunger. Everything tasted great, and I ate it all so I started to gain weight. When I met my wife, I got really happy, and when I'm happy, I eat. Every day was a celebration! We ate like crazy, ordering out pizza, hero sandwiches, or Chinese food all the time. So I gained even more. I used to joke about my weight, which is what a lot of heavy people do to cover up their embarrassment. But in the back of my mind I knew my health situation was real bad, and I was like, "My God, what am I doing?" When I had to go to the doctor for my bus-driving license, he was worried about my weight and high blood pressure and told me to come back for another appointment, but I was scared and never did.

My wife was a Lifetime Member herself, and she was scared for me because by this time I was really heavy. My brothers worried about me, too, and they and my wife would drop hints all the time, but they didn't want to push me. I had kind of an attitude, like, "There's nothing I can do about it so leave me alone!"

Then one day in November 2005 I was putting on my shoes and I got out of breath and had to sit down and rest. That really threw me for a whirl. About two weeks later my brother and I were wrestling, just for fun, and he told me my foot felt puffy. That made me think of my mother, who had been overweight, too, and suffered from swollen feet. She died from congestive heart failure. In a way, my mother saved me—it was like a message from her, telling me I had to change my ways.

So I sat my wife down and told her I wanted to join Weight Watchers. I asked for her help because I knew I couldn't do it alone.

She was 100 percent behind the plan. She was a little concerned because the holidays were coming up, so we decided that I'd just cut back for the next month and wait to join 'til January 7—my birthday—to make it a little bit of a celebration.

I drive a bus into Manhattan and back for New Jersey Transit, so I have to leave around four in the morning. Here's what I used to eat: I'd have a bacon and egg sandwich on the way to the garage, then get some candy from the machine. Once I got to New York, I'd buy a couple of scones. Back in the Jersey garage, I'd have a hero sandwich or take-out Chinese for lunch. When I got home, I'd try to talk my wife into ordering out because I loved the huge quantities of take-out food. If we cooked in, it would always be pasta—I'm Italian and pasta is my life—and I'd go back and fill my plate up three times.

My wife totally blows my mind—she does everything for me, everything! Now she packs me a breakfast to eat in the car on the way to the garage in the morning—usually fruit. Before I get on the bus, I have another piece of fruit. For lunch she packs me a cold-cut sandwich on whole-wheat bread or pita and a salad, with all the parts separated so they won't get soggy, and the dressing on the side. And she keeps me snacking all day so that I'm not hungry: Jell-O, rice cakes, pudding, or low-calorie snack cakes. For dinner, we pretty much stick to pasta, but now it's whole-wheat pasta with just some olive oil and parmesan, and she has this trick where she puts a layer of broccoli under the pasta so that it looks like it's way more than it is. I still go back three times, but there's always the broccoli under the pasta to fill me up.

> "For dinner, we pretty much stick to pasta, but now it's whole-wheat pasta with just some olive oil and parmesan, and she has this trick where she puts a layer of broccoli under the pasta so that it looks like it's way more than it is."

That's not all. She also records all of my **POINTS** for me in my journal and makes sure I get the right amount of oils and dairy. She even keeps a drawer in the kitchen filled with healthy snacks and goodies, so that I don't have to figure it out myself. Of course, I still love food, and every now and then at the garage I'll see people eating like I used to, and I think of my mother and my nana and all the pasta I grew up eating. But in the end I know that being thin and feeling good is better.

I started exercising, too. I began by running around the garage at work—each time around is half a mile. Some people at the garage kind of made fun of me at first, but that didn't bother me—I fed off that negativity. I told myself, "There ain't no way I'm not winning this battle!" My biggest challenge was probably joining the gym because I was afraid I'd get scared and quit. Sure enough, my first day in there, after I signed the papers, I wanted to leave. I always thought that gym people had a certain attitude, and I felt like a stranger in a strange land there. I asked the manager for my money back, and he said, "I can't; you already signed the contract." Well, that guy helped me tremendously, and today he has my before-and-after pictures hanging on the wall. These days, I go after work and do four miles on the treadmill, then all the machines that have to do with the stomach. I think I look okay now. I'm 5 feet 8 inches and getting more toned all the time. I'm working on my six-pack—I'm at four right now—but I'm not interested in looking like a muscleman. I just want to be healthy.

My family is totally involved. After every meeting, my wife would ask me all about it. We've been married seventeen years—it's just the two of us; we don't have kids—but we never had any hobbies together. Now staying fit is our hobby. We sit at the table after dinner and talk about new recipes or new products that are coming out. We take walks together now, and we just bought tennis rackets. We have a whole new life together.

After my meetings, I would also call my older brother and tell him how I was doing. I still do that, and now he's a member, too, so he tells me all about his progress. I'm the baby in the family, the youngest of four brothers, and they've always spoiled me. They pulled for me during my weight loss, and they make a tremendous deal out of me now that I've kept it off for going on two years. When I reached my goal, they had a party, and my brother wrote me a note saying, "Tracy, you achieved the impossible." I'm sorry my mother isn't here to see this because she started it all.

TAKE-AWAY: Ask for support everywhere you can
Be specific and tell family members or friends what they can do to support or assist you as you head toward your goals.

On Becoming a Superhero

Greg Grunberg, 40, California, actor, musician

A while back, I lost a bunch of weight on a no-carb, high-protein, high-fat diet—but the second I reintroduced carbs, the weight came back. When I saw myself in the pilot of *Heroes*, I was like, "Wow." That was my wake-up call.

That and the fact that I had no chin. My clothes didn't fit. I looked bloated and uncomfortable. At the time, I was going through some stressful stuff—and I was eating for comfort. Yet when I saw myself onscreen, I knew I had to do something. My wife, Elizabeth, mentioned WW—and at first, I said I couldn't do it. The last thing I wanted was to sit around calculating **POINTS**. I know it sounds stupid, but I also thought of WW as a women's program. When I checked out the Web site, I was surprised to find a whole section called "eTools for Men," which even mentioned things like beer and pizza! So I decided to try WW. Six months later, I'd dropped 28 pounds. In eight and a half months, I've lost a total of 34 pounds.

And the truth is I hate working out, but I know I have to make time for it. When I'm shooting, I work a twelve-hour day. I'm usually home by 7 p.m. I hang out with my boys, read to them, and then put them to bed by 8:30. By the time I do all that, I'm too tired to work out! I'm not as disciplined as Jennifer Garner was when we shot *Alias*. That's why I work out in the mornings. I wake up to the sound of my wife on the exercise bike. Some couples battle for the bathroom. We battle for the bike! I do twenty-five minutes of interval cardio training. The morning thing is key. One guy in my meeting was going on a cruise for his honeymoon, and he was freaking out about keeping up his workouts. I said, "Okay, dude. When I go on vacation, I work out first thing in the morning. I don't care if it's just a two-mile walk down the beach." The point? When you torture yourself with an early work-out, you tend to want to eat right and stay on track for the rest of the day. If I don't get a morning workout in at home, I use a jump rope for a half hour on the set. It's absolutely one of the best exercises. I do bunny hops in place—fifty one-legged hops at a time, then I alternate the speed to make it an interval workout.

Initially, I got a little flak from my castmates about being on Weight Watchers—but only for about thirty seconds! In our crew, an electrician and a wardrobe stylist also have those WW pedometers hanging from their waists. We're like an underground Fight Club. Any grief I might catch is offset by the fact that thousands of men have been successful on the Program.

Before my weight loss, my big foods were grilled cheese or any kind of pastry. I'm a breadaholic! Chocolate-chip croissants are my kryptonite. If you put a croissant on the end of a fishing rod, I'd follow you anywhere. That's how you can take this Hero down!

> "Chocolate-chip croissants are my kryptonite. If you put a croissant on the end of a fishing rod, I'd follow you anywhere. That's how you can take this Hero down!"

In fact, the *Heroes* producers actually liked the fact that I was overweight! We have all these drop-dead gorgeous people on the show, and I play the Everyman—a relatable cop who is frustrated with his life. I wanted to build my weight loss into the character's story between the first and second seasons. I thought, "Wouldn't it be great if this cop goes through not just a professional and emotional change, but also a physical transformation?" When the producers noticed I was losing weight, they said, "Don't go too far with it." Since the twenty-two episodes happen over twenty-two consecutive days, they were concerned that it would appear that my character had lost 34 pounds in twenty-two "TV days"! But I didn't care. For the first time in my life, I felt educated. For me, the Core Plan is like Weight Watchers University. My family just went to a steakhouse to celebrate my wife's birthday. I looked at the menu and asked, "Which steak has the least amount of marbling?" Then I did something I never would've done before: I split a petit filet with my wife. We butterflied the thing! I learned that portion control tactic from a woman who attends my WW meeting. She cuts everything in half, even her hors d'oeuvres.

Right now, my favorite TV snack break food is celery sticks with yogurt cheese pressed into them. The cheese is low-fat, flavorful, and you can get it at the health-food store. I'm a big cheese guy. I'm also a light beer guy—only two **POINTS**.

TAKE-AWAY: Exercise first thing in the morning

Getting in a workout before the official start of your day helps to ensure that you make time for exercise—and beginning the day in such a healthy way can inspire you to stay on track with your eating all day long.

From Husky
to Marathon Runner

Carlos, 38, Washington, D.C., Realtor

When I was a kid, there were emergency phone numbers on our refrigerator—and Carlos's diet. I was always chubby, and when I was ten or eleven, my pediatrician put me on a diet. My family is Cuban, and healthy cooking was not a part of my mother's repertoire. She would make fried steak with yellow rice and mariquitas, which are fried yucca chips, or fried pork chunks with white rice, black beans, and fried plantains—delicious food but not exactly healthy. We also got rewarded with food whether we were happy or sad. My mom worked at a factory and would get home late so I'd snack in front of the TV after school. A snack would be a grilled ham and cheese sandwich and an industrial-size bag of Doritos. Eating and TV became my best friends. We were copartners in bad habits, which sent me down a bad path with my weight.

I always hated the start of the new school year because I'd have to go shopping for new school clothes. I remember going to the kids' section of the department store, and none of the pants on the rack would fit me. It always ended the same way: the salesperson would announce over the intercom to the stockroom to bring out the husky pants. It was the most humiliating thing! By the time I was in college, my fraternity brothers nicknamed me "Pillsbury," as in the Pillsbury Doughboy, for being the fattest pledge in the class. I hated it! There were so many other things they could have called me, and they picked the one thing I was most upset about, which was my weight. After college I tried my best to lose weight, and sometimes I had some success, but it never lasted.

In 2005, I was changing jobs—from being a full-time fund-raiser to being a Realtor—and I'd gone to the doctor for a physical because of the change in health insurance. The doctor told me I had high blood pressure, high cholesterol, and diabetes. She asked whether I remembered when my parents had developed high blood pressure, and I did because I had to learn how to take my mom's pressure. My mom was fifty-six; she's now almost eighty. When I told the doctor, she said, "Carlos, you're thirty-six. I don't think you'll make it to eighty because your mom had twenty years more before she had to start taking medication." That shocked me. She said that before she put me on medication, she wanted me to lose some weight.

"My meeting leader, Melvin, told me not to think about how far I had to go but to think about losing 1 pound each week. So I put that in my PDA and made that my goal. I started to really focus on making better choices about the foods I put in my mouth."

On my own, I started to eat lighter foods and cut down on portions, and I lost 25 pounds. Then, in October 2005, right before my birthday, the doctor said I definitely had to go on medication. I went to lunch with a friend and I told him that I was really depressed about having to take pills. He said that he was having similar issues and that his mom, who was a member of Weight Watchers, was encouraging him to go. That night, we went together. By then, I was carrying 227 pounds on my 5-foot-7-inch frame.

My meeting leader, Melvin, told me not to think about how far I had to go but to think about losing 1 pound each week. So I put that in my PDA and made that my goal. I started to really focus on making better choices about the foods I put in my mouth. I love to snack so now I always have a bowl of fruit out, and there's always a bag of carrots, a bag of broccoli, and a bag of cauliflower in the fridge. I keep a box of low-fat crackers in the back of my car and a drawer of healthy snacks in my office. I used to come home every night and sit and watch TV. I don't do that anymore because I realized that one of the things I used to do while I sat and watched TV was eat. Now my partner, Michael, and I will go out for a walk after dinner. Gradually, I changed the not-so-healthy habits into healthy habits, and I realized, Oh my God, I can do this! I can really do this!

Six months into it, I really started to see a difference. I had lost 45 pounds, and I was concerned about having sagging skin. A friend of mine who is a personal trainer told me the best way to deal with that was to do calisthenics. Because I had been an overweight kid, I hated sports and I was always bad at them. My friend asked whether I'd tried since I lost weight, and I hadn't so I thought I'd give exercise a try. I started doing a combination of power-walking, lifting light weights, and doing Pilates and other muscle-toning exercises. I got a pedometer and counted my steps, aiming for ten thousand steps a day. Then I began running and walking for fifteen minutes a day on the treadmill, and, gradually, I did it for longer and longer. I never thought I could do this, but last January I did the Miami marathon—and I ran all 26.2 miles!

I've lost almost 70 pounds, and I feel great. I've transformed my life—I have become a kid again. I feel like I'm twenty years old. Not long ago, I had a physical and my doctor said to me, "Carlos, if I didn't know you were almost forty, I'd think you were in your early twenties." There was no evidence of high blood pressure, high cholesterol, diabetes—nothing!

I now feel like I can accomplish anything. What sealed the deal for me was being able to run that marathon. I never saw myself as an athlete before—and now I do. But the best thing about being thinner is the person I see in the mirror every day. In the past, I felt cute but never sexy—and now I do. I still pinch myself every day to see if this is really me.

TAKE-AWAY: Push yourself to get out of your comfort zone

As you're slimming down, make an effort to try new activities that you wouldn't have tried when you were heavier. Discovering how much you enjoy new experiences will bolster your resolve to keep up the good work.

Give Yourself an Oil Change

So much about losing weight involves the choices you make about the food you eat. Jot down a list of several easy, healthier changes or substitutions you can make in your day-to-day eating habits, like switching from butter or oil to vegetable spray. Keep adding to the list as you introduce new foods into your eating plan.

_____

_____

_____

_____

_____

_____

_____

_____

_____

_____

_____

_____

CHAPTER 9

The Power of Teamwork

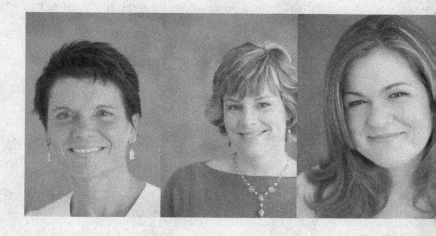

t's been said that no man or woman is an island—and that's also true in the pursuit of life-altering goals. But did you know that when it comes to losing weight or getting fit, doing it with a friend, a family member, or a group increases your sense of personal accountability? In the following stories, men and women share their experiences of losing weight with a spouse, a friend, a family member, or a group of people. They describe how their weight-loss buddies kept them on track and supported them when challenges threatened to derail their efforts. By the end of this chapter, you'll realize how you can harness the power of partnership to help yourself and your pal.

Making Each Other Stronger

Sharon, 66, Illinois, retired pediatric nurse

Gail, 57, Illinois, retired teacher

Sharon: I'm a breast cancer survivor. In 2005, it was my fifth year of being cancer-free, and I realized that I didn't have any more excuses: I was still fat. I had been overweight my whole life. It never seemed to bother my husband, but it was bothering me. I knew I needed a goal, and my good friend Gail's daughters were getting married a year from then. I wanted to look good for the wedding, and I knew Gail did, too, because she'd put on weight. I just called her up and told her I was going to do it. We started Weight Watchers on June 21, 2005.

Gail: I had put on quite a lot of weight after I got married, then I had two children and I kept putting on weight. I went to Europe in June 2005, and when I got my pictures back, I wasn't happy about how I looked—round, puffy, and frumpy. I had my daughter's wedding coming up, then it turned into two weddings because my daughters decided to have a double wedding. So Sharon and I joined together.

Sharon: I think we picked each other to do this because we have totally different personalities. Gail is determined. She is a straight-line walker. I'm a curve. I knew that if I asked Gail to do this, she would never give up and I needed her to make me stronger. We've been friends for thirty-five years.

Gail: I'm a perfectionist by nature. If I made one mistake, I would think that I failed and Sharon would say, "It's just another day" or "You don't throw away twenty-five good things you did because you did one thing that wasn't so good." We drove together to the meetings, and we worked out together at the YMCA four or five times a week. At 8:30 a.m. I'd be in her driveway to pick her up.

Sharon: I liked to sleep until ten o'clock so when I saw her in my driveway, I knew I had to go. We complemented each other, and we knew what buttons to push to keep each other going.

Gail: I think the twenty-minute drive to our meetings and the Y was key because we could talk to each other about our weight struggles, challenges, and triumphs, and get it out of our systems. We would choose when to enjoy life, and we just kept getting closer through the weight-loss experience. I think we were very successful. After belonging to Weight Watchers for about a year, I'd lost a total of 80 pounds and reached my goal. It took Sharon a year and a half to reach her goal.

Sharon: I was able to express that I needed Gail to tell me that I looked better. For a long time, I had stopped looking at myself from the neck down. After I recovered from the cancer, I finally stared into the mirror and thought, "I don't want to look this way in my casket!"

Gail: As we got into smaller sizes, we went shopping together.

Sharon: Gail came up with the idea of giving ourselves presents when we reached our goals. She bought herself new underwear at Victoria's Secret. I had my eyebrows done.

Gail: The biggest goal we were working toward was the wedding. I didn't want to be remembered as the fattest woman there, as the fat mother, since I was going to be one of three mothers in a double wedding. I have to say: I looked awesome. I wore a long pink dress that was fitted at the waist and had some subtle beading around the neck, with a jacket. I felt good!

Sharon: When Gail walked down the aisle, people were like "Whoa!" I got choked up because she looked *that* good. People were so shocked to see us together, looking that good.

Gail: While we were losing weight, because of Sharon's having had breast cancer, some people pulled her husband aside and asked, "Is she okay?" When they found out that she was, they were happy for her that she was losing weight.

Sharon: All told, I lost 82 pounds. My doctors had said they didn't want me to go too low—if I did happen to get sick again, they wanted me to be a little bit rounder, to have some extra reserves to draw from if need be. But we all realized I would never be a size 4. I'm a size 12 now, and that's perfectly comfortable for me. I'm very content and happy with my size now because this is how I can live the rest of my life, and I don't have to think about every single thing I put in my mouth.

One of my biggest compliments came when my husband and I were having dinner out. I'd ordered lemon meringue pie, and I decided that I didn't need to eat the whole thing. I would eat only half of it. The woman who was serving us asked whether I was finished and I said yes. She said, "You know, that's how you thin people stay thin!" I took that as a huge compliment—that she thought I'd always been thin. For me, the best thing about losing weight was becoming what I consider a normal person. To start out as a size 18 and work down to a 12 was just awesome.

> "For me, the best thing about losing weight was becoming what I consider a normal person. To start out as a size 18 and work down to a 12 was just awesome." —Sharon

Gail: I'm a size 10 or 12 now, and I plan to stay this size and be healthy the rest of my life. The numbers are good—my blood pressure and cholesterol have gone down—and I have a whole different feeling about myself. I can go places and do things I never could do before. I now go swimming—I used to hide from swimsuits—and I ride my bike. And last spring Sharon and I completed the 5-K Susan G. Komen Walk for the Cure in St. Louis.

Sharon: There were sixty-five thousand people there in ninety-degree heat, and Gail and her daughters were beside me. It was the first time I tried the whole three miles. At one point, I was having a hard time, but I was so determined. I just kept thinking about putting one foot in front of the other on that yellow line in the road—and I made it. I finished!

Gail: When Sharon stood under the lights with her pink rose at the finish line, it was a marvelous triumph because she never could have done it before losing weight.

TAKE-AWAY: Be realistic

To set yourself up for success in the weight-loss department, aim to achieve a weight that's realistic and healthy for you, given your stage of life, your health, your activity level, and other facets of your life.

Teaching Us How to Take Care of Our Bodies

Teresa, 36, Mississippi, elementary school principal

Carol, 50, Mississippi, assistant principal

Nancy, 48, Mississippi, secretary

Lois, 59, Mississippi, counselor

Lisa, 42, Mississippi, secretary

Teresa: We are trying to be a healthy school. I'm the principal, and those of us in the office—me, the assistant principal, the two secretaries, and the counselor—are basically the face of the school, so it's important for us to present to the public that we do care about ourselves, that we do eat right. The parents like what we're doing because they know the kids are watching us so we are trying to become better role models for their children. In 2005, our school received a $100,000 grant to improve the health of our students and staff, and in January 2007 we started a Weight Watchers meeting at the school for the staff. Out of eighty staff members, thirty-six have joined, and in the first half of 2007 we lost a total of 815 pounds! Those of us in the office lost 135 pounds.

Carol: Everyone at the school is aware of what we're doing because we post our weight loss on the office door every week. We all help one another with sticking to the program and staying healthy. Our music teacher likes to bake muffins for the whole school, and she sends kids around to deliver them. Now when the kids come around, they won't even come into the office—they'll stop right at the door and say, "Oh, you can't have any of this, can you?" The first time that happened, it struck me that what we were doing was hitting home with the kids. You don't have to be an educator long to learn that children notice everything, and that's why it's so important for us to be healthy role models for them.

Nancy: That's true. These kids are in school eight hours a day, some of them longer, and not all of them have healthy role models at home. They look at us to see what we're doing; they really do. School isn't just about book learning, it's also about teaching children to be good stewards of their time, bodies, everything. The teachers usually eat with their students, so that's one way they can model good eating habits.

Carol: Then the kids go home and tell their parents about it, and soon the whole community, the whole town, knows about what we're doing! It's been a big buzz. I've lost weight so my appearance has changed a lot, and when I go around town, to church, to the grocery store, the ball game, people stop me and ask, "What's this program you're doing at the school? Can I join, too?" I really had no idea when we started this that it was going to be such a big deal!

Lois: Several of the teachers who are on the program take their classes to walk laps around the building at lunch or on breaks. That way, they can get their walking in and the kids get to exercise, too. Some of the students used to balk at it, but now they sense the difference in the teachers and they're really getting into it. If one of them sits out the first lap, he or she always joins in by the second.

Nancy: Another thing we've done is put a water machine in the gym, with big bottles of water for 50 cents. And we set a rule that the kids could drink the water anywhere, anytime, even in the classroom. Now these kids drink so much water, it's not even funny! We are all about more activity, more water, less chocolate, less salty and sugary snacks. Although we are very happy about our success with weight loss, around the kids we call it "Eating healthier." We want them to focus on making better choices for life, not on appearances. You have to be very careful about your choice of words with children—they notice everything.

Carol: It's a sad thing, but childhood obesity is a very serious issue not just for our school, but for the whole state of Mississippi. The way we have to combat that is by walking the walk. We'd been focusing on health at our school for a few years—for instance, we started a health class two years ago. But we can't tell the kids to be healthy and then continue to walk around doing unhealthy things ourselves! So by starting the Weight Watchers program, we're trying to show that we're making better choices, too. There was barely a staff member here who didn't need to lose some weight.

Teresa: We are all about taking care of one another. With the grant money, we've set up a fitness room that both kids and staff use, and since the program started, the staff time in the room has almost doubled. We also have a massage therapist come in and offer massages for staff at only $20 per session—and anyone who loses 5 percent or more of his or her body weight gets one for free! We're trying to send the message, to kids and adults alike, that food should never be used as a reward or withheld as a punishment, either. The exercise and massages increase energy levels among the teachers, and they need that—it takes a lot of energy to take care of fourth and fifth graders!

> "You don't have to be an educator long to learn that children notice everything, and that's why it's so important for us to be healthy role models for them."— Carol

Lois: I am the elder of the group, and besides losing weight, I've seen a lowering of my cholesterol and blood pressure, which is wonderful. But for any age, the weight loss and exercise are excellent for stress reduction. We've all seen an improvement in our minds and attitudes. The teachers feel better and are better able to relate to the students. And, of course, there's been a reduction in absenteeism.

As a counselor, I credit it to the group process. Because so many people at our school are doing it, it's like the whole school is one big support group, and that makes us accountable to one another all day long. If I cheat, I'm letting all the other staff members down, and I'm letting the kids down, too. I use this as an opportunity to talk to the kids about making healthy choices—I'll say, "I fought my weight my whole life, and I'm glad I'm doing this now, but I wish I had started when I was your age." And I encourage them to take the message home to their brothers and sisters. I even had one student tell me that she's gotten her mom to come out walking with her. We want to set a good example, and that helps to keep us from backsliding.

> "We're trying to send the message, to kids and adults alike, that food should never be used as a reward or withheld as a punishment, either." — Teresa

Lisa: I've been working here for thirteen years, and it's always been a fun place to work, but since we started the program, it's gotten even better. Losing weight together has pulled us together and we're a lot closer now. What worked for me with this group was being able to ask for help anytime. So I'll come into school and say, "Okay, I'm going out for Mexican food tonight, tell me what I can eat!" Also, I know that walking does wonders for my body, but I really need some kind of encouragement, especially after working all day. Seeing the teachers use the fitness room in our school on their break periods or doing laps around the school really gives me the extra motivation I need.

Teresa: I need motivation to get active, too. Lois was one of the first to start exercising, and that really inspired me. With the stresses of being a first-year principal, plus having young kids at home, it's difficult to find the time. It's been hard telling my husband and kids every morning that I'm going out walking and it doesn't matter what y'all have going on, but I need time to take care of myself. As women, it's important to remember that, and we all help one another.

Nancy: We all help one another in different ways. Behind my desk I have a whole cabinet of low-calorie, low-fat snacks. So when people need something, they just come in and ask. They call me the "Grocery Store"! Just the other day Teresa came in and said, "I'm dying, I need something, but I don't want to blow it!" So I found something to keep her going.

Carol: And having the cafeteria staff on the program is great for everyone, too, because it's forcing them to think about the fat and sugar content of the foods they cook for us. The other day our cafeteria manager came in and said, "I just cooked squash for the school lunch for the first time, y'all!" We can go to her and ask, "What's healthy today?" and now she knows! And, of course, that's something that's affecting the kids, too, because she'll be able to steer the kids toward healthier choices. Another thing Teresa and I were talking about is maybe setting up a sort of fruit sale for the kids, the way some schools have vending machines or bake sales. Maybe a kind of farmers' market right in school!

At the end of last year, the PTO—that's like our PTA—threw us a teacher-appreciation party, and they served salsa and vegetables, and healthy sandwiches, and low-cal cakes topped with strawberries. That meant a lot to us.

Teresa: This year, the annual Mississippi Department of Education's Mega Conference, in Biloxi, invited us to attend and present what we've done with staff wellness and health education in general here at Grenada. Besides the Weight Watchers program, we've taken out all soda machines and made the school lunches healthier; we started measuring students' BMIs [body mass index, an indication of whether someone is overweight]; and our school nurse is going to begin working with students whose BMIs are high. We're also really uncomfortable with the tradition of selling chocolate bars to raise money, so we're replacing those with fruit snacks and peanuts. And we're seeing results with the kids. We've definitely noticed fewer sodas, more water, and more baked, rather than fried, chips in the lunches they bring from home. I can't tell you how proud we are of ourselves and of what we're doing for the kids. We really hope that they will take these messages home with them, pass them on to their own families, and end up making a change for the whole state of Mississippi.

TAKE-AWAY: Check in with your support system regularly

Talking with people you trust about challenges you face can help you to keep things in perspective and stay on track as you pursue your goals.

A Couple's Journey to a Better Life

Kathy, 56, Florida, human resources director for an HMO

Bill, 58, Florida, systems safety director for an HMO

Kathy: Two years ago, Bill and I were coming up on our thirty-fifth anniversary. We wanted to celebrate by going to Alaska, but when you're as heavy as we were, there was no way we could fit comfortably in the seats on a plane. I had flown a couple of times for business, and it was very uncomfortable and embarrassing. I'd have to ask for a seat-belt extender, and I'd worry that even if the person sitting next to me was a normal size, I'd be over on his or her seat.

Bill: And I didn't fly at all because of my weight.

Kathy: Really, our initial incentive to lose weight was that we needed to drop some pounds so that we could fit into the seats on the plane. But there were a lot more reasons to lose weight, of course.

Bill: The health aspect was big, but our main goal was to feel better. If we lost weight, our knees wouldn't hurt, and we wouldn't be out of breath when we were walking. In my spare time, I'm a skeet shooter. The field is only about forty yards long, and I used to be huffing and puffing by the time I got around it.

Kathy: I would walk in from the parking lot to my job and have to stop to catch my breath. I had had open-heart surgery when I was eighteen, and I knew the shortness of breath wasn't good for my ticker. Also, we have a beautiful six-year-old granddaughter and we wanted to be able to do things with her, like take her to Disney World.

Bill: Growing up, I was always big—and bigger than other kids, but I didn't think about my weight. In high school I played on the football team.

Kathy: As a child, I was thin, but everything seemed to change after the heart surgery, and then gaining weight was a gradual process. I didn't see myself as that heavy, until I started not being able to do things like fit into the seat at a movie theater.

For many years, I simply didn't pay attention to myself. My mother had a stroke when she was forty-two and I was seventeen. I took care of her pretty much my whole adult life, sometimes full time, sometimes part time. I was stressed out and a caregiver, plus working, and a mother to two kids. My eating habits had really gotten out of control.

My mother passed away two weeks before I joined Weight Watchers. I had always done something with her on Thursday nights, so I joined on a Thursday night—March 17, 2005. I've lost 96 pounds.

Bill: When Kathy joined, I said I'd follow along with the program. I told her, "You put the food in front of me, and I'll eat it." By the time I actually joined on December 31, 2005, I'd already taken off a good amount of weight—over 80 pounds from my top weight of 388, and I hadn't set foot in a meeting yet. What happened was, we stopped in one morning for Kathy to weigh in. I was so amazed at how motivational the leader was that I joined on the spot. I'm now 241 pounds. My goal is 208.

The excess weight had been putting constant pressure on my knees. It got to the point where my doctor had prescribed a souped-up ibuprofen, the only thing that took the edge off. When I lost the weight, I got rid of that medication. And now I can do the whole round of a skeet field without worrying about my breathing.

Kathy: When we were heavier, we wouldn't socialize much at skeet competitions. We'd just sit in the background. The other weekend, though, I stepped up and helped with meal preparation, and one of the girls said to me, "Not only have you and Bill changed with your weight, the biggest change is that you've come out of your shell. You're sociable, and you talk. When you were heavier, you were quieter, you weren't approachable." I hadn't meant to be that way, but when I was heavier, I wanted to stay out of sight. I guess we both felt inferior.

Bill: When you're overweight, it's like living in a shell, like a tortoise getting away from danger. I used to go into my shell to get away from people. People looked at us differently. I'd catch them out of the corner of my eye, shaking their heads. I didn't want to see that. They'd give us negative looks, and I was sure they were thinking, "Why'd you let yourself go? You're ugly."

Kathy: People kept telling us that we both looked great after losing weight but that the biggest difference was that it's really fun to be around us. For our part, we had a good time and enjoyed people's company that weekend at the skeet competition.

Life is a lot better in so many ways. When we go out to eat, now we ask for a booth—we don't want a table because to us a table represents being heavy; you can move a chair out, but you can't move a built-in bench. Now we go out and walk and go places without thinking about how far it is or whether our knees will hurt. We're not afraid to walk up hills. We both walk a lot more, and I've started water aerobics. But we could both benefit from more exercise. We need to firm up—when you lose that kind of weight, you become flabby in a lot of areas.

> "When we started losing the weight, we got rid of the bigger-size clothes. It's cost us a fortune over the two years! But if we had kept the clothes, it would have been as if they were giving us permission to put the weight back on."
> — Kathy

When we started losing the weight, we got rid of the bigger-size clothes. It's cost us a fortune over the two years! But if we had kept the clothes, it would have been as if they were giving us permission to put the weight back on—and we didn't want that to fall back on.

Bill: The best thing about being thinner is staying out of the big and tall shops, being able to buy clothes in a regular store. I've gone from a size-60 to a size-42 waist. I kept one pair of big jeans. When I hit my goal weight, I'm going to wear them to a meeting. I'll probably have to tie 'em with a rope! It's been a heck of a journey. I'm not on a diet; I'm on a journey to better health and a better life.

Kathy: Now that we're thinner, we plan on traveling a lot more than we did before. For our thirty-fifth anniversary, we made it to Alaska, which is such a beautiful, beautiful state. Not only did we have a wonderful time, we're planning to go back next summer for two weeks.

TAKE-AWAY: Think of things you'd want to do if your weight weren't an issue

Whether you want to go sailing, learn to salsa, or travel to faraway places, keep in mind activities you've longed to try but haven't because of your excess weight. This will provide a built-in incentive to slimming down.

A Ton of Inspiration

Emilie, 52, Delaware, radiology customer service coordinator for a medical center

Nancy, 50, Delaware, community relations specialist for public relations

Peggy, RN, MSN, 48, Delaware, clinical education specialist

Jeanne, RN, 63, Delaware, employee health nurse

Barbara, RN, 52, Delaware, nursing instructor and Weight Watchers leader

Jeanne: As health-care workers—our medical center is a community hospital with a school of nursing and nearly sixteen hundred employees—we know we should lead healthy lifestyles, but unfortunately we don't always do that. There are many who smoke, who don't exercise, who overeat. One problem is that people who work in hospitals work all different shifts—weekends and nights—so it's not always easy to stick with regular, healthy dietary or exercise habits. We live in a small town, and some of the gyms near us aren't open when we are able to go. Nurses traditionally work twelve-hour shifts, and sometimes, by the end of a shift, we're tired and we don't have the energy to get to a fitness center, even if it is open. And it's not as beneficial to exercise after you've worked a twelve-hour shift—it's better to go when you're not exhausted.

Barbara: We know what we should do, but it's another challenge to alter our behaviors and do the right thing. We're just as susceptible to not listening to ourselves as our patients are!

Jeanne: And things change. I'd always been able to manage my weight. I exercised and tried to watch what I ate. Then, when I turned sixty, I put on 10 pounds. When I turned sixty-one, I put on another 10 pounds. As I hit sixty-two, I added 5 more. When I realized I was about to go into a size 12, I knew I needed to do something. Weight Watchers was already under way here, and I went with a coworker. I won't say I went kicking and screaming, but I kind of felt like I did. And then that first week I lost weight, which I hadn't been able to do. Now I'm a believer. I joined in the spring of 2006.

Emilie: I was a very skinny kid who never ate anything—that is, until I went to college, where I gained the freshman 15 and didn't stop. I had two kids and just kept putting on the weight. When I got to be about forty-five, I developed high blood pressure. The doctors kept saying that if I lost weight, my cholesterol and blood pressure would go down.

Barbara: I was *never* the skinny kid—I was always the fat kid. You name a diet, I've done it. I would lose and gain back, lose and gain back. I joined Weight Watchers in 2004 and lost 103 pounds from my top weight of 231.

Nancy: When you're heavy, it affects your knees. I've been able to postpone knee surgery because I've lost weight. I've had seven knee surgeries, so not to have another one means a lot. And even though I went through the death of my mother, whom I took care of, last year, I didn't gain anything. I'm proud of that. I needed something that was regimented to keep me on track.

Barbara: The At Work program got started after I went to the regular Weight Watchers meeting and lost my excess weight. When everyone started asking, "Oh my gosh, what did you do?!" Jeannie and I had a powwow and I suggested bringing Weight Watchers in. Jeannie is very pro-health for our employees and she went for it.

Jeanne: When I started, I heard stories like Emilie's—people who were able to go off blood pressure medicine or avoid diabetes medications because of their weight loss. Then our VP of human resources joined, and she started to hear the same stories. She decided that reimbursement might encourage more people to join, so now employees are reimbursed for up to three twelve-week sessions, as long as they attend 75 percent of the meetings, not just get weighed in, and make progress.

Barbara: We started the Weight Watchers program here in February 2006. Just six months later, the health-care costs for our first thirty or so members—for lab work, doctor visits, X-rays, tests, and procedures of these types—had gone down $43,000. And all of us together have lost 2,456 pounds—more than a ton!

Jeanne: We're concerned with more than just weight. The employee health department has a walking program called the 1,000-K club, which has been in place for ten or fifteen years. People do it together. They grab one another and say, "Hey, let's go for a walk." People have various excuses not to work out—they can't afford to belong to a gym; they don't have time—but with this, they can easily go walking on a break or at lunchtime. There's a 1-K loop right outside the hospital.

Barbara: During the meetings I push for people to join the 1,000-K club since exercise is a critical part of any weight-loss journey.

Emilie: Many of us exercise at home, too. I have a lab puppy who requires lots of walks. I do half a mile in the morning and half a mile at night, seven days a week. I can talk a person out of walking, but I can't talk the dog out of walking! I have so much more energy these days since I'm walking, have shed extra pounds, and am eating a more balanced diet. I used to go to bed at nine o'clock every night. I'm able to stay up 'til ten o'clock now and do things like cleaning when I get home from work, rather than sitting down and watching TV.

> "I have so much more energy these days since I'm walking, have shed extra pounds, and am eating a more balanced diet." —Emilie

Peggy: I like to go to the boardwalk or the beach to walk. I try to do it at least three times a week.

Barbara: I walk, and my husband and I do distance bicycling, anywhere from twenty-five to seventy-five miles a shot!

Emilie: Another thing that's great is meeting people from the school of nursing. There's at least 150 people who have done Weight Watchers, and we've gotten to know one another.

Jeanne: When I was a staff nurse, I knew no one but the nurses on my shift. Through the At Work meetings, we get to know people who work in the OR, in our foundation, in medical records. I do believe it's boosted morale and given us a sense of camaraderie. Our support system is critical, especially during stressful times and the holidays.

Emilie: During Christmas season, we donated our treats to Barb and she distributed them elsewhere, so that we weren't eating them here or taking food home. She also sent our Girl Scout cookies—the ones that Peggy didn't eat!—to the soldiers in Iraq.

> "I've lost weight and have been able to postpone knee surgery because of it. I've had seven knee surgeries, so not to have another one means a lot." —Nancy

Peggy: Cookies are my weakness.

Barbara: My son happened to be there at the time, and I was able to send three big boxes of cookies. So the employees didn't have to feel guilty—we still bought them from the cute little girls, but we didn't eat them.

Emilie: We have one cafeteria, open from eleven to one. You see Weight Watchers people there all the time. In my department, I became—by agreement—the **POINTS** guru. I would tell them how many **POINTS** they were eating and whether they were eating healthy or not.

Peggy: One of the tough things is there's always food around. Whatever you're doing, people are bringing in bags of chips and candy, and everyone keeps munching. I also work in the emergency department and patients' families often bring food in for us as a thank-you.

Nancy: One thing I found out is that when you are going through a tough time and having trouble staying on the program, you have a support system right at work. Sometimes the hardest time is when you're headed to the cafeteria, but then you see people there and you can work out food problems together.

Jeanne: For instance, one of my coworkers will often suggest splitting a dish if something looks good but is a huge portion. Or, sometimes we'll be in the cafeteria and nothing appeals. But someone will be sure to suggest a hamburger or a chicken breast off the grill—without the bun—and they'll know how many **POINTS** it is, too.

Barbara: We help one another all the time. I received an e-mail the other day titled "Weight Watchers 911." When I opened it up, it was someone asking, "How many **POINTS** are in cheesecake, STAT! We need to know." I answered the question, and then the person was able to make a good choice: not to eat that cheesecake.

Nancy: It's nice to have that support system around you all the time.

Barbara: When you work in a place with sixteen hundred people, it's easy not to know them. Hospitals are notorious for staying with our own "towers" or work groups. I migrate to nurses in the cafeteria, and it's the same with lab or radiology people. Your HR department might plan a picnic for the whole place, and I can promise you that the lab people will huddle together, the nurses will huddle together, the radiology people will huddle together. But all of us trying to lose weight together has broken that apart. Now I might migrate to radiology or lab people in the cafeteria, not just nurses. When you have people stepping out to say hi to others, the whole workplace gets more positive and pleasant. And it enhances communication in the organization. For example, if I have a patient issue, I can talk more easily to Emilie because I already know her. I never knew Emilie before. I had missed this beautiful person, and because of Weight Watchers I got to meet her. She's touched my life, and we'll never forget each other. It's a bonus I didn't expect.

TAKE-AWAY: Donate sweets to a worthy cause
When fund-raisers come around, with people selling cookies, candies, or other confections, buy as many packages as you'd like and donate them to a charitable organization that will distribute them to people who'd appreciate them. That way, you won't feel guilty about not supporting the cause—or about eating the goodies.

A Mother and Daughter Losing It Together

Kaye, 52, Tennessee, certificate processor for an insurance broker

Alicia, 32, Tennessee, retail operations administrator for a bank

Kaye: I had just had a physical with a new doctor, and my blood pressure was high. He said I had to lose weight by my next appointment, or he was going to put me on medication. I weighed 194 pounds. I wasn't surprised by his reaction because I had battled my weight my entire adult life—the result of a diet heavy on fried foods and no portion control. I could eat twelve cookies without even blinking. I'd been on and off a number of diets before I joined Weight Watchers in March 2005, shortly after my physical. After I'd been on the plan for a month or so, I called my daughter Alicia, who lives about an hour away, and told her how well it was working.

I admit, I had an ulterior motive when I called her. Alicia was quite overweight, but I had never said anything to her about it because I knew that I felt resentful and angry when anyone said anything to me about my weight. I didn't want to do anything to harm our relationship. But I was secretly hoping that she'd want to try the program, too.

Alicia: I was totally in denial about my weight. I'd had three kids in four years, and I gained 30 pounds with each one, but I never admitted to myself that I was overweight. I wore maternity clothes for almost four years straight, and I never weighed myself. No one ever mentioned my weight to me, so I just let myself go on thinking I was fine.

The trouble was, I was having lots of back pain, and I had been for a few years. I'd been to the doctor many times and had lots of tests, but they couldn't find anything wrong. It was so bad I could hardly sleep at night. One night I actually went to the emergency room, and they gave me morphine for the pain, but they still couldn't find anything wrong. When my mom told me that Weight Watchers was working for her, I thought it might be worth a try. My belly was pretty big, and I thought it might be putting a strain on my back. I joined in June 2005, and I was completely surprised when I stepped on the scale at my first meeting. I weighed 237 pounds! That's a huge number, especially for someone who's 5 feet 5 inches. It sounds crazy, but I was obese and didn't even realize it.

Kaye: I was so relieved when Alicia joined because I'd been quite worried about her health, and I could finally talk to her more openly about her weight. No one likes to hear that they're overweight, and it's especially hard for a daughter to hear it from her mother. But what really surprised me was how much more motivated I felt to stick with the program after she joined. There's nothing worse for a mother than watching her child suffer. I wanted her to be out of pain and to be a healthy weight, and I knew that the best way to help her was to stick with the program myself. Doing it with her and for her helped me to stay focused.

Alicia: I e-mailed Mom every single week after my meeting. I loved to tell her I'd lost weight because I knew she'd be proud of me. And if I didn't lose weight, the e-mail gave me a chance to analyze what went wrong. Maybe I didn't drink enough water or I slacked off on my exercise. Knowing that Mom was out there rooting for me helped me to stay on track even when I felt like I didn't want to do it anymore. If I had a moment of weakness, I'd tell myself, "You can't let Mom down."

Kaye: Of course, we also e-mailed each other about any new foods we heard about in our groups, like the kettle corn we both like, and some recipes, like a chicken and rice dish. I was really excited when Alicia told me she had started to prepare healthier foods for her children. Alicia had grown up eating fried, fatty foods because that was my diet, and I know this played a role in her weight problem. So I was happy that she was turning the tables for my grandchildren. Her middle child loves broccoli now.

Alicia: My kids have learned to eat healthier, thanks to my new diet.

I always serve a vegetable and a fruit with every meal. We have lots of salads, and the kids love them. I don't want my kids to let their weight get out of control because taking it off is hard—it's better never to gain in the first place. I did well for the first six months, and I was really motivated because my back started to feel a lot better. Then I hit a plateau. I'd go up a pound and down a pound. I started walking a little more and changed what I was eating, and the scale finally started to move again.

Kaye: My weight loss went more smoothly than I would have imagined. My blood pressure went to normal almost as soon as I started to lose, and I gave myself rewards for reaching small goals—I bought new down pillows when I lost my first 10 pounds. After that, I realized I didn't need a reward because the weight loss was a reward in itself. It was just so nice to look in the mirror and see a slimmer person, and my clothes looked better on me. I thought it would be fun for Alicia to have something to look forward to, so I told her that when she reached her goal weight, I'd buy her a new wardrobe. I hit my goal of 141 pounds on January 3, 2006, on my thirty-first wedding anniversary. I was so excited, I called Alicia from my meeting.

> "My kids have learned to eat healthier, thanks to my new diet. I always serve a vegetable and a fruit with every meal. I don't want my kids to let their weight get out of control because taking it off is hard—it's better never to gain in the first place." —Alicia

Alicia: I couldn't believe it. I was so happy for her—and I couldn't wait to join her in success. But I had a way to go. Finally, I reached my goal of 150 in March 2007, and we celebrated by buying me a new wardrobe. I got a black suit in a size 10—a size I hadn't worn in years.

My husband recently showed me a picture of what I looked like before I lost weight, and I was in shock. I still can't believe I let myself get that big. Even though I weigh the same now as I did in college, I feel slimmer than I ever have, and I feel so much healthier, too. Before, I was always tired. I thought it was because I had three little kids, but I see now that it was because of my weight. I feel like I'm a better mom. I can play at the park, I can ride a bike, I can get down on the ground and play with my kids. I couldn't do any of that before.

Kaye: I feel like I'm a better mom, too. I had unintentionally contributed to Alicia's weight problems by teaching her unhealthy eating habits, and then I let it go on by not mentioning her weight gain to her. Now I've helped her break those bad habits and helped her back pain go away. Nothing could be more gratifying than that—not even losing weight myself.

TAKE-AWAY: Don't hide underneath your clothes

Wearing baggy outfits may feel more comfortable when you're overweight, but they can keep you in denial about your weight. It's better to wear clothes that fit well to remind you of your long-term diet and fitness goals—and of the slimmer you that you want to be.

Go Public with Your Goals

When you tell trusted friends and family members about your commitment to lose weight, you're more likely to stick with it because you'll want others to see you following through. Who are your current biggest supporters and who are potential supporters to help you along the way?

_____

_____

_____

_____

_____

_____

_____

_____

_____

_____

_____

_____

Credits

Photographer, Maura McEvoy; hair and makeup stylist, Sara Johnson; wardrobe stylist, Sarah Parlow

Cover models: Top, left to right: Fran (story on page 56), Nicola (story on page 127), Carlos (story on page 203), Lisa (story on page 38); bottom, left to right: Joseph (story on page 53), Sandy (story on page 99), Bettyann (story on page 178), Jane (story on page 154)

Interior models (left to right): Page 9: Sara (story on page 47), Monica (story on page 123); page 63: Sandra (story on page 65), Rolando (story on page 190); page 89: Susan (story on page 113), Melissa (story on page 94)

Index

CPSIA information can be obtained
at www.ICGtesting.com
Printed in the USA
LVHW030249040121
675576LV00004BA/1051

9 781620 455715